# ABC OF
# ANTITHROMBOTIC THERAPY

# ABC OF
# ANTITHROMBOTIC THERAPY

Edited by

## GREGORY Y H LIP

*Professor of cardiovascular medicine and director, haemostasis, thrombosis and vascular biology unit, university department of medicine, City Hospital, Birmingham*

*and*

## ANDREW D BLANN

*Senior lecturer in medicine, haemostasis, thrombosis and vascular biology unit, university department of medicine, City Hospital, Birmingham*

First published in 2003
Second impression in 2003

by BMJ Publishing Group Ltd, BMA House, Tavistock Square,
London WC1H 9JR

www.bmjbooks.com

**British Library Cataloguing in Publication Data**
A catalogue record for this book is available from the British Library

ISBN 0 7279 17714

Typeset by BMJ Electronic Production and Newgen Imaging Systems
Printed and bound in Spain by GraphyCems, Navarra

Cover image depicts a deep vein thrombosis scan of a leg vein blocked by a thrombus (blood clot, white)
in a patient with deep vein thrombosis. With permission from James King-Holmes/Science Photo Library

# Contents

# Contributors

**Andrew D Blann**
Senior lecturer in medicine, haemostasis, thrombosis and vascular biology unit, university department of medicine, City Hospital, Birmingham

**Bernard S P Chin**
Research fellow, haemostasis, thrombosis and vascular biology unit, university department of medicine, City Hospital, Birmingham

**Derek L Connolly**
Consultant cardiologist, department of cardiology and vascular medicine, Sandwell and West Birmingham Hospitals NHS Trust, Sandwell Hospital, West Bromwich

**Dwayne S G Conway**
Research fellow, haemostasis, thrombosis and vascular biology unit, university department of medicine, City Hospital, Birmingham

**David A Fitzmaurice**
Reader in primary care and general practice, Medical School, University of Birmingham, Edgbaston, Birmingham

**Ira Goldsmith**
Research fellow in cardiothoracic surgery, haemostasis, thrombosis and vascular biology unit, university department of medicine, City Hospital, Birmingham

**Robert G Hart**
Professor of neurology, department of medicine (neurology), University of Texas Health Sciences Center, San Antonio, USA

**Bernd Jilma**
Associate professor in the department of clinical pharmacology, Vienna University Hospital, Vienna, Austria

**Sridhar Kamath**
Research fellow, haemostasis, thrombosis and vascular biology unit, university department of medicine, City Hospital, Birmingham

**Martin J Landray**
Lecturer in medicine, haemostasis, thrombosis and vascular biology unit, university department of medicine, City Hospital, Birmingham

**Gregory Y H Lip**
Professor of cardiovascular medicine and director, haemostasis, thrombosis and vascular biology unit, university department of medicine, City Hospital, Birmingham

**Andrew J Makin**
Research fellow, haemostasis, thrombosis and vascular biology unit, university department of medicine, City Hospital, Birmingham

**Neeraj Prasad**
Consultant cardiologist, City Hospital, Birmingham

**Stanley H Silverman**
Consultant vascular surgeon, City Hospital, Birmingham

**Alexander G G Turpie**
Professor of medicine, McMaster University, Hamilton, Ontario, Canada

**Robert D S Watson**
Consultant cardiologist, City Hospital, Birmingham

# Preface

The seeds for this book were sown with the establishment of the haemostasis, thrombosis and vascular biology unit at the university department of medicine, City Hospital, Birmingham—with the coming together of clinicians and scientists interested in thrombosis and vascular biology, bridging the previous divide in thrombosis between basic science research and the application to clinical practice. Indeed, thrombosis is the underlying pathophysiological process in a wide variety of conditions. A greater understanding of the mechanisms leading to thrombosis, and newer developments in the field of antithrombotic therapy make the field all the more dynamic and exciting.

The multidisciplinary team effort and the wide range of research areas studied in our unit forms the core content of the *ABC of Antithrombotic Therapy*. In major textbooks on thrombosis the scope is comprehensive, background details on physiology and pathophysiology are abundant, and treatment options are listed to exhaustion—the patient may sometimes almost disappear in the wealth of information. Our approach in this book—typical of the ABC series in the *British Medical Journal*—tries to synthesise and integrate the extensive research and clinical data that are needed to manage a particular situation as masterly as it is possible. We hope we have produced a patient-oriented guide with relevant information from clinical epidemiology, pathophysiology, common sense clinical judgement, and evidence based treatment options, with reference to recently published antithrombotic therapy guidelines from the American College of Chest Physicians, British Society for Haematology, European Society of Cardiology, American College of Cardiology, and American Heart Association.

Our expectant readers are physicians, general practitioners, medical or nursing students, nurses, and healthcare scientists who care for patients presenting with thrombosis-related problems, and thus, the scope is necessarily wide, ranging from venous thromboembolism to atrial fibrillation and stroke, and to thrombosis in cancer and thrombophilic states. Chapters on clinical pharmacology and bleeding risk, as well as anticoagulation monitoring are included. Furthermore, this book includes additional chapters which were not included in the 14 issues of this series when it first appeared in the *British Medical Journal*.

We thank our excellent colleagues for their help, encouragement and contributions, as well as Sally Carter at BMJ Books for encouraging us to complete the series and book, nearly to schedule.

Gregory Y H Lip
Andrew D Blann
Birmingham, April 2003

# 1 An overview of antithrombotic therapy

Andrew D Blann, Martin J Landray, Gregory Y H Lip

Many of the common problems in clinical practice today relate to thrombosis. The underlying final pathophysiological process in myocardial infarction and stroke is thrombus formation (thrombogenesis). Common cardiovascular disorders such as atrial fibrillation and heart failure are also associated with thrombogenesis. Thrombosis is also a clinical problem in various cancers and after surgery, especially orthopaedic.

## Pathophysiology

Over 150 years ago Virchow recognised three prerequisites for thrombogenesis: abnormal blood flow, vessel wall abnormalities, and blood constituent abnormalities. This concept has been extended by modern knowledge of the endothelial function, flow characteristics, and blood constituents including haemorheological factors, clotting factors, and platelet physiology. As thrombus consists of platelets and fibrin (and often bystanding erythrocytes) optimum antithrombotic prophylactic therapy can and should be directed towards both.

## Antiplatelet drugs

**Aspirin and agents acting on the cyclo-oxygenase pathway**
Aspirin irreversibly inhibits cyclo-oxygenase by acetylation of amino acids that are next to the active site. In platelets, this is the rate limiting step in synthesis of thromboxane $A_2$, and inhibition occurs in the megakaryocyte so that all budding platelets are dysfunctional. Because platelets are unable to regenerate fresh cyclo-oxygenase in response, the effect of aspirin remains as long as the lifespan of the platelet (generally about 10 days). A severe weakness of aspirin is that its specificity for cyclo-oxygenase means it has little effect on other pathways of platelet activation. Thus aspirin fails to prevent aggregation induced by thrombin and only partially inhibits that induced by ADP and high dose collagen. Antithrombotic doses used in clinical trials have varied widely from less than 50 mg to over 1200 mg/day, with no evidence of any difference in clinical efficacy. Absorption is over 80% with extensive presystemic metabolism to salicylic acid. Only the parent acetylsalicylic acid has any significant effect on platelet function.

*Adverse effects* of aspirin include haemorrhage, hypersensitivity and skin rashes, alopecia, and purpura.

Sulfinpyrazone also inhibits cyclo-oxygenase (thus producing an aspirin-like state), but is reversible, and also inhibits serotonin uptake by platelets. Iloprost is a prostacyclin analogue that exerts its effects by promoting vasodilatation and inhibiting platelet aggregation induced by ADP, thereby opposing the effects of thromboxane $A_2$.

**Dipyridamole**
Dipyridamole inhibits phosphodiesterase, thus preventing the inactivation of cyclic AMP, intraplatelet levels of which are increased, resulting in reduced activation of cytoplasmic second messengers. However, it may also exert its effect in other ways, such as stimulating prostacyclin release and inhibiting thromboxane $A_2$ formation. The influence of this drug on these pathways causes reduced platelet aggregability and adhesion in

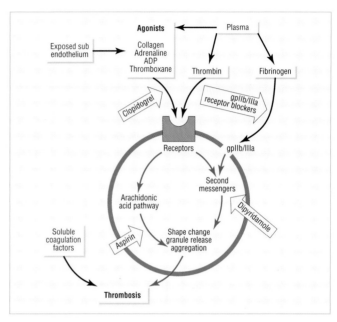

Routes to inhibiting platelet function

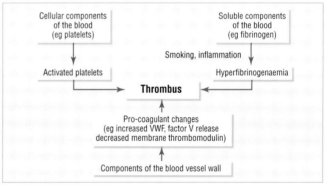

Key components of Virchow's triad (VWF=von Willebrand factor)

**Contraindications to aspirin**

| Absolute | Relative |
|---|---|
| ● Active gastrointestinal ulceration | ● History of ulceration or dyspepsia |
| ● Hypersensitivity | ● Children over 12 years old |
| ● Thrombocytopenia | ● Bleeding disorders |
| | ● Warfarin treatment |

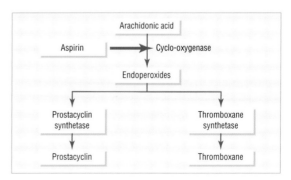

Platelet metabolism influenced by aspirin

vitro with increased platelet survival in vivo. Its effect is relatively short lasting, and repeated dosing or slow release preparations are needed to achieve 24 hour inhibition of platelet function.

### Clopidogrel and ticlopidine
These thienopyridine derivatives inhibit platelet aggregation induced by agonists such as platelet activating factor and collagen, and also dramatically reduce the binding of ADP to a platelet surface purinoreceptor. The mechanism of this inhibitory action seems to be independent of cyclo-oxygenase. There is also impairment of the platelet response to thrombin, collagen, fibrinogen, and von Willebrand factor. The peak action on platelet function occurs after several days of oral dosing. Adverse effects include evidence of bone marrow suppression, in particular leucopenia, especially with ticlopidine.

### Other receptor blockers
Signal transduction generally occurs when specific receptors on the surface are occupied by ligands such as ADP, leading to structural modification of the glycoprotein IIb/IIIa receptor on the surface of the platelet. This is the commonest receptor on the platelet surface and represents the final common pathway for platelet aggregation, resulting in crosslinking of platelets.

After intravenous administration of glycoprotein IIb/IIIa receptor inhibitors such as abciximab, platelet aggregation is 90% inhibited within two hours, but function recovers over the course of two days. The major adverse effect is haemorrhage, and concurrent use of oral anticoagulants is contraindicated. Eptifibatide is a cyclic heptapeptide that mimics the part of the structure of fibrinogen that interacts with glycoprotein IIb/IIIa. Thus it is a fraction of the size of abciximab and is targeted at the same structure on the platelet surface.

Clinical trials with oral glycoprotein IIb/IIIa receptor inhibitors have been disappointing, with no beneficial effects seen and even some evidence of harm.

# Anticoagulant drugs

### Warfarin
This 4-hydroxycoumarin compound, the most widely used anticoagulant in Britain and the Western world, inhibits the synthesis of factors dependent on vitamin K (prothrombin; factors VII, IX, and X; protein C; protein S). Factor VII levels fall rapidly (in < 24 hours) but factor II has a longer half life and only falls to 50% of normal after three days. Warfarin is approximately 97% bound to albumin, and free warfarin enters liver parenchymal cells and is degraded in microsomes to an inactive water soluble metabolite that is conjugated and excreted in the bile. Partial reabsorption is followed by renal excretion of conjugated metabolites.

There is a considerable variability in warfarin's effect on patients, its effectiveness being influenced by age, racial background, diet, and co-medications such as antibiotics. Thus it demands frequent laboratory monitoring, the prothrombin time being compared with a standard to produce the international normalised ratio. The degree of anticoagulation required varies with clinical circumstance, but the target international normalised ratio usually ranges from 2 to 4. Phenindione is an alternative oral vitamin K antagonist, but concerns regarding the potential for hepatotoxicity, nephrotoxicity, and blood dyscrasias have reduced its role largely to individuals with documented hypersensitivity to warfarin.

*Adverse effects* of warfarin include haemorrhage, hypersensitivity and skin rashes, alopecia, and purpura.

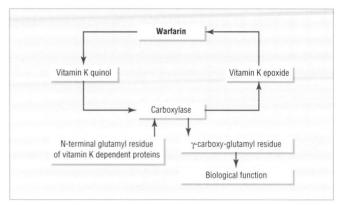

Vitamin K metabolism and the effect of warfarin

---

### Factors that influence the efficacy of warfarin*

#### Patient factors
- *Enhanced anticoagulant effect*—Weight loss, increased age (> 80 years), acute illness, impaired liver function, heart failure, renal failure, excess alcohol ingestion
- *Reduced anticoagulant effect*—Weight gain, diarrhoea and vomiting, relative youth (< 40 years), Asian or African-Caribbean background

#### Examples of drug interactions with warfarin
- *Reduced protein binding*—Aspirin, phenylbutazone, sulfinpyrazone, chlorpromazine
- *Inhibition of metabolism of warfarin*—Cimetidine, erythromycin, sodium valproate
- *Enhanced metabolism of warfarin*—Barbiturates, phenytoin, carbamazepine
- *Reduced synthesis of factors II, VII, IX, X*—Phenytoin, salicylates
- *Reduced absorption of vitamin K*—Broad spectrum antibiotics, laxatives
- *Enhanced risk of peptic ulceration*—Aspirin, NSAIDs, corticosteroids
- *Thrombolytics*—Streptokinase, tissue plasminogen activator
- *Antiplatelet drugs*—Aspirin, NSAIDs

*This list is intended to be illustrative not exhaustive

---

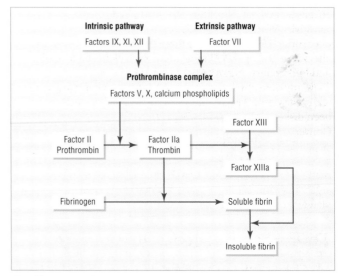

Simplified coagulation cascade

## Melagatran

This oral thrombin inhibitor undergoing phase III trials seems to be well tolerated, with few clinically significant bleeding problems, in patients with venous thromboembolism. Although considerable pharmacokinetic and animal data exist, solid evidence of its effectiveness compared with warfarin and heparin in patients at high or low risk is still awaited.

## Heparin

Heparin is a glycosaminoglycan whose major anticoagulant effect is accounted for by a pentasaccharide with a high affinity for antithrombin III. This binding results in a conformational change in antithrombin III so that inactivation of coagulation enzymes thrombin (IIa), factor IXa, and factor Xa is markedly enhanced. Its short half life means it must be given continuously, and its extensive first pass metabolism means it must be given parenterally, preferably by continuous intravenous infusion, and it is therefore inappropriate for home use. The effect on the intrinsic clotting cascade must be monitored carefully by measuring the activated partial thromboplastin time (APTT), generally aiming for a value 1.5 to 2.5 times that of control.

Unfractionated heparin consists of a heterogeneous mixture of polysaccharides with an average molecular weight of 15 000 Da. Low molecular weight heparins (4000-6000 Da) are weaker inhibitors of thrombin but inhibit factor Xa to a similar extent. Different commercial preparations of low molecular weight heparin vary in the ratio of anti-Xa to antithrombin activity, although the clinical relevance of this is uncertain. Better absorption after subcutaneous administration and reduced protein binding result in greatly improved bioavailability. The effective half life after subcutaneous injection is four hours, allowing an injection once daily in most circumstances. These more predictable pharmacokinetics allow the dose to be calculated on the basis of the patient's weight and reduce the requirement for frequent monitoring. In those rare cases where monitoring is deemed necessary, measurement of plasma levels of anti-Xa activity is needed. Tests of APTT are unhelpful.

*Major adverse effects* of heparin include haemorrhage, osteoporosis, alopecia, thrombocytopenia, and hypersensitivity. At present, the risk of haemorrhage seems to be similar with low molecular weight and unfractionated heparin. However, the risk of heparin induced thrombocytopenia seems to be less with the low molecular weight form.

## Hirudin and direct thrombin inhibitors

Hirudin, a 65 amino acid residue anticoagulant peptide with a relative molecular mass of 7000 Da purified from the leech *Hirudo medicinalis*, binds thrombin with high specificity and sensitivity. With a true half life of about an hour and a half life effect on the APTT of two to three hours, it may be seen as an alternative to heparin in indications such as unstable angina and in coronary angioplasty.

Many derivatives are available, with hirulog and argatroban among the best developed. However, trials of the former have been discouraging: no clear benefit over heparin was shown. Conversely, argatroban may have a role in the anticoagulation of patients unable to tolerate heparin as a result of heparin induced thrombocytopenia. Furthermore, in a clinical trial of patients with heparin induced thrombocytopenia, use of argatroban was associated with a reduction in levels of plasma platelet activation markers.

# Thrombolytic agents

These agents lyse pre-existing thrombus, either by potentiating the body's own fibrinolytic pathways (such as streptokinase) or

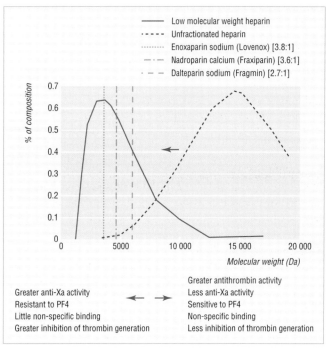

The three low molecular weight heparins that have been evaluated in clinical trials of acute coronary syndromes are shown with their respective anti-Xa and antithrombin activity (PF4=platelet factor 4)

**Comparison of low molecular weight and unfractionated heparins**

| | Unfractionated heparin | Low molecular weight heparin |
|---|---|---|
| Action | Anti-XIIa, XIa, IXa, VIIa, antithrombin | Mostly anti-Xa |
| Route of administration | Subcutaneous Intravenous | Subcutaneous |
| Absorption from subcutaneous route | Slow | Improved |
| Protein binding | Proteins in plasma and on endothelium | Reduced |
| Bioavailability | Subcutaneous—10-30% at low doses, 90% at higher doses Intravenous—100% by definition | >90% |
| Effective half life | Subcutaneous—1.5 hours Intravenous—30 min | 4 hours |
| Between and within individual variation | Extensive | Minimal |
| Monitoring | APTT | Not required (anti-Xa activity) |
| Elimination | Liver and kidney | Kidney |

# ABC of Antithrombotic Therapy

by mimicking natural thrombolytic molecules (such as tissue plasminogen activator). The common agents in clinical use are derived from bacterial products (streptokinase) or manufactured using recombinant DNA technology (recombinant tissue plasminogen activator). Newer drugs aim to be less antigenic and more thrombus specific in an attempt to increase efficacy and specificity of various agents; on present evidence, however, the differences between thrombolytic agents are only marginal. Because of the lack of site specificity for these drugs, the major adverse effect is that of haemorrhage (gastrointestinal, intracranial, etc). The other important adverse effect is that of hypersensitivity reaction, especially with streptokinase. This usually manifests as flushing, breathlessness, rash, urticaria, and hypotension. Severe anaphylaxis is rare. Hypersensitivity reactions are avoided by using tissue plasminogen activator or recombinant tissue plasminogen activator, which are not antigenic.

## Streptokinase

Derived from streptococci, this product is an effective thrombolytic agent for the treatment of acute myocardial infarction and pulmonary thromboembolism. Acting by converting plasminogen to plasmin, the main fibrinolytic enzyme, it potentiates fibrinolysis. However, it is not site specific, lysing thrombus anywhere in the body. Being bacteria derived, it is antigenic, and repeated administration results in neutralising antibodies and allergic reactions. For example, a single administration of 1.5 MU for acute myocardial infarction results in neutralising antibodies that have been shown to persist for up to four years and are sufficient to neutralise a repeat administration of a similar dose of the agent in half of cases.

## Tissue plasminogen activator

In clinical use this is produced by recombinant DNA technology and mimics an endogenous molecule that activates the fibrinolytic system. Thus, recombinant tissue plasminogen activator does not elicit an allergic response and is considered more clot specific. Nevertheless, it has a short half life and needs continuous infusion to achieve its greatest efficacy. Accelerated administration of tissue plasminogen activator gives a slight mortality advantage over streptokinase at the cost of a marginal increase in stroke rate.

### Fibrinolytic drugs

| Examples | Source | Mechanism of action |
| --- | --- | --- |
| Streptokinase | Group C β haemolytic streptococci | Complexes with and activates plasminogen |
| Urokinase | Trypsin-like chemical produced by kidney | Direct acting plasminogen activator |
| Reteplase (recombinant tissue plasminogen activator) | Recombinant DNA technology | Acivates plasminogen, non-immunogenic |

### Contraindications to thrombolysis

**Absolute**
- Recent or current haemorrhage, trauma, or surgery
- Active peptic ulceration
- Coagulation defects
- Oesophageal varices
- Coma
- Recent or disabling cerebrovascular accident
- Hypertension
- Aortic dissection

**Relative**
- Previous peptic ulceration
- Warfarin
- Liver disease
- Previous use of anistreplase or streptokinase within four years (use alternative agent)
- Hypersensitivity (anistreplase, streptokinase)
- Heavy vaginal bleeding

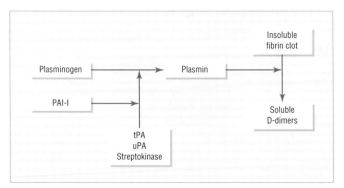

Simplified fibrinolysis (PAI-1=plasminogen activator inhibitor, tPA=tissue plasminogen activator, uPA=urokinase plasminogen activator)

## Further reading

- Antiplatelet Trialists' Collaboration. Collaborative overview of randomised trials of antiplatelet therapy, I: Prevention of death, myocardial infarction, and stroke by prolonged antiplatelet therapy in various categories of patients. *BMJ* 1994;308:81-106
- Blann AD, Lip GYH. Virchow's triad revisited: the importance of soluble coagulation factors, the endothelium, and platelets. *Thromb Res* 2001;101:321-7
- CAPRIE Steering Committee. A randomised, blinded, trial of clopidogrel versus aspirin in patients at risk of ischaemic events (CAPRIE). *Lancet* 1996;348:1329-39
- Catella-Lawson F. Direct thrombin inhibitors in cardiovascular disease. *Coron Artery Dis* 1997;8:105-11
- Eriksson H, Eriksson UG, Frison L. Pharmacokinetic and pharmacodynamics of melagatran, a novel synthetic LMW
- thrombin inhibitor, in patients with a DVT. *Thromb Haemost* 1999;81: 358-63
- International Stroke Trial Collaborative Group. The international stroke trial (IST): a randomised trial of aspirin, subcutaneous heparin, or both, or neither among 19 435 patients with acute ischaemic stroke. *Lancet* 1997;349:1569-81
- Lewis BE, Wallis DE, Berkowitz SD, Matthai WH, Fareed J, Walenga JM, et al. Argatroban anticoagulant therapy in patients with heparin-induced thrombocytopenia. *Circulation* 2001;103:1838-43
- Nurden AT. New thoughts on strategies for modulating platelet function through the inhibition of surface receptors. *Haemostasis* 1996;20:78-88
- Stirling Y. Warfarin-induced changes in procoagulant and anticoagulant proteins. *Blood Coagul Fibrinolysis* 1995;6:361-73

The figure showing percentage of composition of unfractionated and low molecular weight heparin in terms of molecular weight is adapted from Levine GN, Ali MN, Schafer AI. *Arch Intern Med* 2001;161: 937-48.

# 2 Bleeding risks of antithrombotic therapy

David A Fitzmaurice, Andrew D Blann, Gregory Y H Lip

Many of the common cardiovascular disorders (especially in elderly people) are linked to thrombosis—such as ischaemic heart disease, atrial fibrillation, valve disease, hypertension, and atherosclerotic vascular disease—requiring the use of antithrombotic therapy. This raises questions regarding the appropriate use of antithrombotic therapy in older people, especially because strategies such as anticoagulation with warfarin need regular monitoring of the international normalised ratio (INR), a measure of the induced haemorrhagic tendency, and carry a risk of bleeding. The presence of concomitant physical and medical problems increases the interactions and risks associated with warfarin, and anticoagulation in elderly patients often needs an assessment of the overall risk:benefit ratio.

Physical frailty in elderly people may reduce access to anticoagulant clinics for INR monitoring. The decline in cognitive function in some elderly patients also may reduce compliance with anticoagulation and the appreciation of bleeding risks and drug interactions. However, in recent studies of anticoagulation in elderly people, no significant associations of anticoagulant control were found with age, sex, social circumstances, mobility, domicillary supervision of medication, or indications for anticoagulation.

## Warfarin

Bleeding is the most serious and common complication of warfarin treatment. For any given patient, the potential benefit from prevention of thromboembolic disease needs to be balanced against the potential harm from induced haemorrhagic side effects.

### Minor bleeds

Most bleeding problems are clinically minor, although patients are unlikely to view such bleeds in these terms. The problems include nose bleeds, bruising, and excessive bleeding after minor injury such as shaving. Patients should be made aware of these common problems and be reassured that these events are expected in patients receiving warfarin treatment. Menorrhagia is surprisingly rare as a major clinical problem, even though it can be severe.

### More serious problems

Patients need access to medical care if they have serious problems. Such problems are generally due to a high INR. Usually, spontaneous bruising, any bleeding that is difficult to arrest, frank haematuria, any evidence of gastrointestinal bleeding, and haemoptysis, need urgent assessment. The definition of minor or major bleeding lacks clarity: in many cases the patient presents with a concern that may need follow up, and a minor bleed can only be defined as such in retrospect. In most cases, evidence of bleeding suggests some underlying pathology but may also be due to drug interactions. For example, a patient with recurrent haemoptysis may be found to have hereditary telangectasia. Further investigation of the cause of bleeding should always be considered, particularly if the bleeding is recurrent. It is also important in these instances to check for concomitant drug use, particularly drugs received over the counter. Patients should be aware that aspirin and

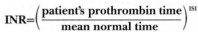

**Questions to ask when considering oral anticoagulation**
- Is there a definite indication (such as atrial fibrillation)?
- Is there a high risk of bleeding or strong contraindication against anticoagulation?
- Will concurrent medication or disease states increase bleeding risk or interfere with anticoagulation control?
- Is drug compliance and attendance at anticoagulant clinic for monitoring likely to be a problem?
- Will there be regular review of the patient, especially with regard to risks and benefits of anticoagulation?

$$INR=\left(\frac{\text{patient's prothrombin time}}{\text{mean normal time}}\right)^{ISI}$$

**ISI=international sensitivity ratio. The mean normal prothrombin time is often generated from samples from local healthy subjects or a commercially available standard. The exact value of the ISI depends on the thromboplastin used in the prothrombin time method**

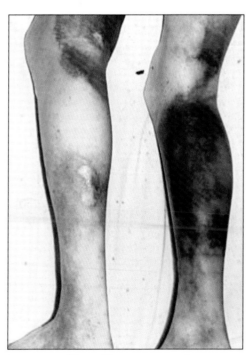

Purpura, petechiae, and haematoma secondary to over-anticoagulation

**Sudden, unexplained changes to the efficacy of warfarin may be caused by the consumption of over the counter multivitamin tablets or foodstuffs that contain high levels of vitamin K**

non-steroidal anti-inflammatory drugs are particularly dangerous in combination with warfarin; however, even supposedly safe drugs such as paracetamol can affect a patient's bleeding tendency.

### Incidence of bleeding problems

The incidence of severe bleeding problems that may bring patients to an accident and emergency unit has probably been overestimated. The annual incidence of fatality caused by warfarin administration has been estimated to be 1%. However, this is based on old data, and, although difficult to prove, the overall improvement in anticoagulation control in the past 10-15 years means that a more realistic figure is about 0.2%. Methodological problems have hampered the interpretation of previously reported data, particularly with regard to definitions of major and minor bleeding episodes, with some investigators accepting hospital admission for transfusion of up to 4 units of blood as being "minor." Certainly, the most serious "major" bleed is an intracranial haemorrhage. Reviews of observational and experimental studies showed annual bleeding rates of 0-4.8% for fatal bleeding and 2.4-8.1% for major bleeds. Minor bleeds are reported more often, with about 15% of patients having at least one minor event a year.

### Risk factors for bleeding

Age is the main factor that increases risk of bleeding. One study showed a 32% increase in all bleeding and a 46% increase in major bleeding for every 10 year increase above the age of 40.

Early studies suggested an increased risk with increasing target INR, but the data were difficult to interpret because results were reported in both INR and prothrombin time. The actual risk of bleeding should be taken into account as well as the degree of anticoagulation (as measured by the INR). One study which achieved point prevalence of therapeutic INRs of 77% reported no association between bleeding episodes and target INR.

Data from an Italian study in 2745 patients with 2011 patient years of follow up reported much lower bleeding rates, with an overall rate of 7.6 per 100 patient years. The reported rates for fatal, major, and minor bleeds were 0.25, 1.1, and 6.2 per 100 patient years respectively. This study confirmed an increased risk with age and found a significantly increased risk during the first 90 days of treatment. Peripheral vascular and cerebrovascular disease carried a higher relative risk of bleeding, and target INR was strongly associated with bleeding with a relative risk of 7.9 (95% confidence interval 5.4 to11.5, P < 0.0001) when the most recent INR recorded was >4.5. Data from a trial in a UK community showed 39.8 minor, 0.4 major, and no fatal haemorrhagic events per 100 patient years for the total study population, with 3.9 serious thromboembolic events per 100 patient years, of which 0.79 were fatal.

Warfarin is therefore a relatively safe drug, particularly if therapeutic monitoring is performed well. Analogies are often made between therapeutic monitoring of warfarin and monitoring of blood glucose for diabetic patients. Given the increase in numbers of patients receiving warfarin, particularly for atrial fibrillation, the scale of the problem is likely to be the same. There is no reason why warfarin monitoring cannot become as routine as glucose monitoring in diabetes: relevant small machines are available for generating an INR (with associated standards and quality control).

### Overanticoagulation

Excessive anticoagulation without bleeding or with only minor bleeding can be remedied by dose reduction or discontinuation. The risk of bleeding is decreased dramatically by lowering the intended INR from 3-4.5 down to 2-3, although this increases

---

**Patients at high risk of bleeding with warfarin**
- Age >75 years
- History of uncontrolled hypertension (defined as systolic blood pressure >180mm Hg or diastolic blood pressure >100 mm Hg)
- Alcohol excess (acute or chronic), liver disease
- Poor drug compliance or clinic attendance
- Bleeding lesions (especially gastrointestinal blood loss, such as peptic ulcer disease, or recent cerebral haemorrhage)
- Bleeding tendency (including coagulation defects, thrombocytopenia) or concomitant use of non-steroidal anti-inflammatory drugs and antibiotics
- Instability of INR control and INR >3

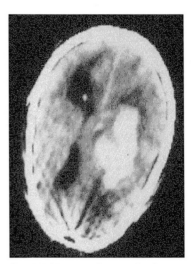

Computed tomography scan showing intracerebral haemorrhage

---

**Risk of bleeding associated with warfarin treatment**
- Rate of bleeding episodes associated in the general patient population is decreasing (possibly due to better management)
- Risk increases with age
- Risk of bleeding is directly related to the achieved intensity of INR rather than the target INR (a clear dose-response effect)
- Temporal association between measured INR and risk of bleeding
- Relative risk of bleeding is increased in patients with cerebrovascular disease and venous thrombosis

the risk of thrombosis. If bleeding becomes substantial, 2-5 mg of oral or subcutaneous vitamin K may be needed. In patients with prosthetic valves, vitamin K should perhaps be avoided because of the risk of valve thrombosis unless there is life threatening intracranial bleeding. Alternatives to vitamin K include a concentrate of the prothrombin group of coagulation factors including II, IX, and X, fresh frozen plasma 15 ml/kg, and recombinant factor VIIa.

# Aspirin

Aspirin has little effect in terms of bruising but can cause serious gastrointestinal bleeding. The risk of gastrointestinal bleeding is related to dose and should not be problematic at doses of 75 mg/day given as thromboprophylaxis. There is currently no consensus as to optimal dose of aspirin for stroke prevention in atrial fibrillation. A meta-analysis of randomised controlled trials using aspirin showed that a mean dose of 273 mg/day, increased absolute risk of haemorrhagic stroke to 12 events per 10 000 people. This relatively small increase must be weighed against the reduced risk of myocardial infarction (to 137 events per 10 000) and ischaemic stroke (to 39 events per 10 000). However, in one trial of patients with well controlled hypertension, use of aspirin 75 mg prevented 1.5 myocardial infarctions per 1000 patients a year, which was in addition to the benefit achieved by lowering the blood pressure, with no effect on stroke. Although there was no increase in the number of fatal bleeding events (seven in patients taking aspirin, compared with eight in the placebo group), there was a 1.8% increase in non-fatal, major bleeding events (129 events in patients taking aspirin, compared with 70 in the placebo group) and minor bleeds (156 and 87, respectively).

# Risk of bleeding

There have been conflicting results concerning the role of age as an independent risk factor for haemorrhage induced by anticoagulants. Advanced age ($>75$ years), intensity of anticoagulation (especially INR $>4$), history of cerebral vascular disease (recent or remote), and concomitant use of drugs that interfere with haemostasis (aspirin or non-steroidal anti-inflammatory drugs) are probably the most important variables determining patients' risk of major life threatening bleeding complications while they are receiving anticoagulation treatment.

Generally elderly people have increased sensitivity to the anticoagulant effect of warfarin, and require a lower mean daily dose to achieve a given anticoagulant intensity. For example, patients aged $>75$ years need less than half the daily warfarin dose of patients aged $<35$ for an equivalent level of anticoagulation. Whatever the mechanism it is clear that warfarin therapy needs careful justification for being given to elderly patients, and the dose needs modification and careful monitoring.

As there is an exponential increase in bleeding risk with a linear increase in anticoagulant effect, there will be a substantial increase in bleeding risk with overanticoagulation. For example, the annual risk of bleeding rises from 1.6% in elderly people not treated with anticoagulant drugs (based on the "Sixty-Plus" study), to 5% (relative risk 3) at an INR of 2.5, and to 50% (relative risk 30) at an INR of 4. In another study, total bleeding events were 39% in a group of 31 patients with an INR of 7 compared with 13% in a group of 100 with a stable INR (odds ratio 5.4, 95% CI 2.1-13.9). The greatest risk factor for being in this group was (apart from having a high target INR) antibiotic therapy in the preceding four weeks.

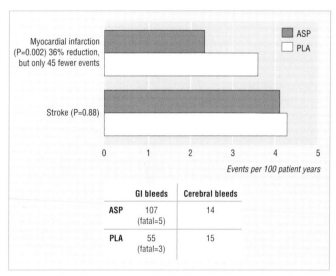

| | GI bleeds | Cerebral bleeds |
|---|---|---|
| ASP | 107 (fatal=5) | 14 |
| PLA | 55 (fatal=3) | 15 |

Myocardial infarction, stroke, and bleeding in the hypertension optimal treatment trial (HOT) study (ASP=aspirin, PLA=placebo)

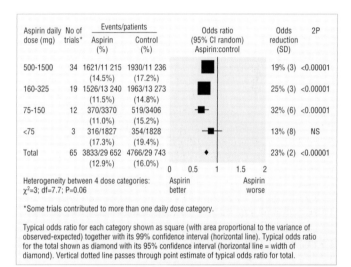

*Some trials contributed to more than one daily dose category.

Typical odds ratio for each category shown as square (with area proportional to the variance of observed-expected) together with its 99% confidence interval (horizontal line). Typical odds ratio for the total shown as diamond with its 95% confidence interval (horizontal line = width of diamond). Vertical dotted line passes through point estimate of typical odds ratio for total.

Effect of different doses of aspirin in secondary prevention of vascular events (There is no significant difference in benefit with different aspirin doses, but at higher doses adverse effects are more likely)

**Variables that may influence the risk of bleeding in elderly people**
- Increased sensitivity to the effect of anticoagulation, perhaps due to increased receptor affinity or lower dietary vitamin K intake
- Concurrent use of drugs that increase bleeding risk
- Associated comorbidity and other diseases that decrease compliance and increase the risk of bleeding

**Possible reasons for increased sensitivity to anticoagulation in elderly people**
- Lower body weight
- Differences in pharmacokinetics, with a tendency towards reduced drug clearance in the elderly either due to decreases in renal or hepatic blood flow and function with age per se or disease processes
- Change in receptor sensitivity
- Lower dietary vitamin K intake in the elderly may perhaps be the more important cause

Multiple drug therapy or polypharmacy is quite common, with the consequence of adverse drug interactions, the risk of which rises exponentially with the number of drugs given simultaneously and with concurrent diseases. Typical drug interactions include changes in absorption across intestinal mucosae and hepatic metabolism. Patients should be cautioned about the risk of warfarin-drug interactions when their medication list is altered. The decline in cognitive function in some elderly patients may mean they do not realise that some drugs can interact with anticoagulants and so they do not mention their use of oral anticoagulants to doctors or pharmacists. However, elderly patients are likely to attend clinic less often than younger patients, suggesting a greater degree of INR stability.

Many diseases associated with stroke and thromboembolism are more common with increasing age. Older patients are often at highest risk, and appropriate anticoagulation therapy reduces morbidity and mortality. Careful and continuing evaluation of patients is necessary to ensure that the risks of bleeding do not outweigh the benefits from anticoagulation.

The diagram showing the results of the hypertension optimal treatment trial is adapted from Hansson L, et al. *Lancet* 1998;351:1755-62. The figure showing the effect of different doses of aspirin in secondary prevention of vascular events is reproduced from *Clinical Evidence* (June issue 7), BMJ Publishing Group, 2002.

## Further reading

- Blann AD, Hewitt J, Siddique F, Bareford D. Racial background is a determinant of average warfarin dose required to maintain the INR between 2.0 and 3.0. *Br J Haematol* 1999;10:207-9
- Erhardtsten E, Nony P, Dechavanne M, Ffrench P, Boissel JP, Hedner U. The effect of recombinant factor VIIa (NovoSeven™) in healthy volunteers receiving acenocoumarol to an International Normalized Ratio above 2.0. *Blood Coag Fibrin* 1998;9:741-8
- Fitzmaurice DA, Hobbs FDR, Murray ET, Hodder, RL, Allan TF, Rose, PE. Oral anticoagulation management in primary care with the use of computerised decision support and near-patient testing. A randomised controlled trial. *Arch Intern Med* 2000;160:2323-48
- Gurwitz JH, Goldberg RJ, Holden A, Knapic N, Ansell J. Age-related risks of long term oral anticoagulant therapy. *Arch Intern Med* 1988;148:1733-6
- He J, Whelton PK, Vu B, Klag MJ. Aspirin and risk of haemorrhagic stroke. *JAMA* 1998;280:1930-5
- Haemostasis and Thrombosis Task Force of the British Society for Haematology. Guidelines on oral anticoagulation: third edition. *Br J Haematol* 1998;101:374-87
- Landefeld CS, Beyth RJ. Anticoagulant related bleeding: clinical epidemiology, prediction, and prevention. *Am J Med* 1993;95:315-28
- Levine MN, Hirsh J, Landefeld CS, Raskob G. Haemorrhagic complications of anticoagulant treatment. *Chest* 1992;102:352-63S
- Panneerselvan S, Baglin C, Lefort W, Baglin T. Analysis of risk factors for over-anticoagulation in patients receiving long-term warfarin. *Br J Haematol* 1998;103:422-4
- Palareti G, Leali N, Coccheri S, Poggi M, Manotti C, D'Angelo A, et al. Bleeding complications of oral anticoagulant treatment: an inception-cohort, prospective collaborative study (ISCOAT). *Lancet* 1996;348:423-8
- van der Meer FJM, Rosendaal FR, Vandenbroucke, Briet E. Bleeding complications in oral anticoagulant therapy. *Arch Int Med* 1993;153:1557-62
- Hutton BA, Lensing AWA, Kraaijenhagen RA, Prins MH. Safety of treatment with oral anticoagulants in the elderly. *Drugs and Aging* 1999;14:303-12

# 3 Venous thromboembolism: pathophysiology, clinical features, and prevention

Alexander G G Turpie, Bernard S P Chin, Gregory Y H Lip

Venous thromboembolism is a common complication among hospital inpatients and contributes to longer hospital stays, morbidity, and mortality. Some venous thromboembolisms may be subclinical, whereas others present as sudden pulmonary embolus or symptomatic deep vein thrombosis. Ultrasonic Doppler and venographic techniques have shown deep vein thrombosis of the lower limb to occur in half of all major lower limb orthopaedic operations performed without antithrombotic prophylaxis. Deep vein thrombosis of the lower limb is also seen in a quarter of patients with acute myocardial infarction, and more than half of patients with acute ischaemic stroke.

Deep vein thrombosis of the lower limb normally starts in the calf veins. About 10-20% of thromboses extend proximally, and a further 1-5% go on to develop fatal pulmonary embolism. Appropriate antithrombotic measures can reduce this complication. Until recently, some clinicians were reluctant to provide such prophylaxis routinely. As unfounded fears of major bleeding complications from anticoagulant regimens wane, preventive treatments are used more often with medical and surgical patients. However, the risk of bleeding can be serious and this has particular bearing in postoperative patients.

Venous thromboembolism can also arise spontaneously in ambulant individuals, particularly if they have associated risk factors such as thrombophilia, previous thrombosis, or cancer. However, in over half of these patients, no specific predisposing factors can be identified at presentation.

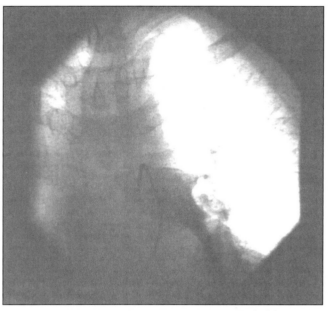

Pulmonary angiography showing large pulmonary embolus in left pulmonary artery

## Pathophysiology

Thrombus formation and propagation depend on the presence of abnormalities of blood flow, blood vessel wall, and blood clotting components, known collectively as Virchow's triad. Abnormalities of blood flow or venous stasis normally occur after prolonged immobility or confinement to bed. Venous obstruction can arise from external compression by enlarged lymph nodes, bulky tumours, or intravascular compression by previous thromboses. Increased oestrogens at pharmacological levels, as seen with oral contraceptive use and with hormone replacement therapy in postmenopausal women, have been associated with a threefold increased risk in the small initial risk of venous thromboembolism. Cancers, particularly adenocarcinomas and metastatic cancers, are also associated with increased venous thromboembolism. Indeed, on presentation, some idiopathic venous thromboembolisms have revealed occult cancers at follow up. Both oestrogens at pharmacological levels and cancer can also activate the clotting system.

## Clinical presentation and diagnosis

### Deep vein thrombosis

Deep vein thrombosis commonly presents with pain, erythema, tenderness, and swelling of the affected limb. Thus, in lower limb deep vein thrombosis, the affected leg is usually swollen with the circumference of the calf larger than the unaffected side. Other causes of leg swelling, erythema, and tenderness include a ruptured Baker's cyst and infective cellulitis. The

> **Venous thromboembolism often manifests clinically as deep vein thrombosis or pulmonary embolism, and is possibly one of the preventable complications that occur in hospitalised patients**

---

**Risk factors and conditions predisposing to venous thromboembolism**

- History of venous thromboembolism
- Prolonged immobility
- Prolonged confinement to bed or lower limb paralysis
- Surgery, particularly lower limb orthopaedic operations, and major pelvic or abdominal operations
- Trauma—For example, hip fractures and acute spinal injury
- Obesity
- Major medical illnesses such as acute myocardial infarction, ischaemic stroke, congestive cardiac failure, acute respiratory failure
- Oestrogen use in pharmacological doses—For example, oral contraception pills, hormone replacement therapy
- Cancer, especially metastatic adenocarcinomas
- Age >40 years
- Aquired hypercoagulable states—Lupus anticoagulant and antiphospholipid antibodies, hyperhomocysteinaemia, dysfibrinogenaemia, myeloproliferative disorders such as polycythaemia rubra vera
- Inherited hypercoaguable states—Activated protein C resistance (factor V Leiden mutation), protein C deficiency, protein S deficiency, antithrombin deficiency, prothrombin gene mutation

---

diagnosis of deep vein thrombosis is therefore more likely when risk factors are present and less so if there are features suggesting alternative diagnoses. For example, ruptured Baker's cysts commonly appear in the context of osteoarthritis and rheumatoid arthritis. Infective cellulitis is unlikely to be bilateral, with clearly demarcated areas of erythema extending proximally. Breaks in the skin, particularly between the toes, and coexistent fungal infection are additional clues to cellulitis.

Objective diagnosis of venous thromboembolism is important for optimal management. Although the clinical diagnosis of venous thromboembolism is imprecise, various probability models based on clinical features have proved to be practical and reliable (interobserver reliability, $\kappa = 0.85$) in predicting the likelihood of venous thromboembolism. These models should be used in conjunction with objective diagnostic tests.

Compression ultrasonography remains the non-invasive investigation of choice for the diagnosis of clinically suspected deep vein thrombosis. It is highly sensitive in detecting proximal deep vein thrombosis although less accurate for isolated calf deep vein thrombosis. In patients with suspected thrombosis and a negative compression ultrasound result, the test should be repeated in seven days because studies have shown that patients with two or more negative tests over a week who are untreated have a less than 2% risk of proximal extension or subsequent deep vein thrombosis.

Impedance plethysmography is slightly less specific and sensitive than ultrasonography but may still have a role in pregnant women and suspected recurrent deep vein thrombosis. The gold standard is invasive contrast venography, which is still used when a definitive answer is needed. Newer imaging techniques are being developed, and tools such as magnetic resonance venography or computed tomography could possibly detect pelvic vein thromboses, but further testing is needed to establish their role in the diagnosis of deep vein thrombosis.

Blood tests such as fibrin D-dimer add to the diagnostic accuracy of the non-invasive tests. In one study, the sensitivity and specificity of a D-dimer concentration of $>500\ \mu g/l$ for the presence of pulmonary embolism were 98% and 39%, respectively, which give positive and negative predictive values of 44% and 98%. The sensitivity of the test even remained high at three and seven days after presentation (96% and 93%).

### Modified pretest probability for deep vein thrombosis

| Clinical feature | Score |
| --- | --- |
| Tenderness along entire deep vein system | 1.0 |
| Swelling of the entire leg | 1.0 |
| Greater than 3 cm difference in calf circumference | 1.0 |
| Pitting oedema | 1.0 |
| Collateral superficial veins | 1.0 |
| Risk factors present: | |
|   Active cancer | 1.0 |
|   Prolonged immobility or paralysis | 1.0 |
|   Recent surgery or major medical illness | 1.0 |
| Alternative diagnosis likely (ruptured Baker's cyst in rheumatoid arthritis, superficial thrombophlebitis, or infective cellulitis) | −2.0 |

Score >3 = high probablility; 1-2 = moderate probability <0 = low probability

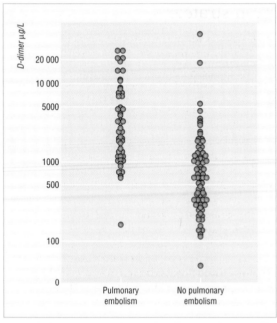

Plasma D-dimer concentrations on day of presentation according to final diagnosis

### Investigations for suspected venous thromboembolism by pretest clinical probability

| Pretest probability | Fibrin D-dimer | Other investigations | Comment |
| --- | --- | --- | --- |
| **Deep vein thrombosis:** | | | |
| Low | Negative | | No further investigations needed |
| Low or moderate | Positive | Negative ultrasound compression | Consider venography or repeat ultrasound after a week |
| Moderate or high | Positive | Positive ultrasound compression | Treat with anticoagulants |
| High | Positive | Negative ultrasound compression | Consider venography to rule out deep vein thrombosis, especially in high risk patients and those with recurrent pulmonary emboli |
| **Pulmonary embolism:** | | | |
| Low | Negative | No | No further investigation needed |
| Low or moderate | Positive | Proceed to ventilation-perfusion scan | If non-diagnostic ventilation-perfusion scan consider serial compression ultrasound over two weeks to rule out venous thromboembolism |
| High | Positive | Proceed to ventilation-perfusion scan (or ultrasound) | If non-diagnostic ventilation-perfusion scans, proceed to venography or pulmonary angiography as needed |

## Pulmonary embolism

Patients presenting with acute pulmonary embolism often complain of sudden onset of breathlessness with haemoptysis or pleuritic chest pain, or collapse with shock in the absence of other causes. Deep vein thrombosis may not be suspected clinically, but its presence, along with thrombotic risk factors, will make the diagnosis of pulmonary embolism more likely. A similar clinical probability model to that for deep vein thrombosis has been developed for pulmonary embolism.

Pulmonary angiography is the gold standard investigation for pulmonary embolism, but it is invasive and associated with 0.5% mortality. A ventilation-perfusion scan using technetium DTPA (ditriaminopentaric acid) is more widely used. However this investigation is non-specific, and is diagnostic in only 30% of cases. Spiral computed tomography scans are more reliable but diagnosis is limited to emboli in larger vessels only. Measurement of fibrin D-dimer levels, used for deep vein thrombosis, is helpful, as is compression ultrasound in the detection of occult deep vein thrombosis.

# Prevention strategies

An appropriate strategy for the prevention of venous thromboembolism include pharmacological or physical methods. To optimise treatment, patients should be stratified into risk categories to allow the most appropriate prophylactic measure to be used.

Prophylactic drugs include unfractionated heparin, low molecular weight heparin, oral anticoagulants (such as coumarins), thrombin inhibitors (such as hirudin), and specific factor Xa inhibitors (such as fondaparinux). The recently approved fondaparinux reduces the risk of venous thromboembolism after orthopaedic surgery by more than half compared with low molecular weight heparin and seems likely to become the treatment of choice after universal availability.

Prophylactic physical methods include the use of compression elastic stockings, intermittent pneumatic compression (which provides rythmic external compression at 35-40 mm Hg for about 10 seconds every minute), and early mobilisation to improve venous blood flow in conditions predisposing to venous stasis.

### General surgery

Patients at low risk undergoing general surgery do not need specific prophylaxis other than early mobilisation. In moderate risk patients, fixed low doses of unfractionated heparin (5000 IU every 12 hours) or low molecular weight heparin (3400 anti-Xa units or equivalent) once daily is sufficient. Higher doses of low molecular weight heparin (more than 3400 IU anti-Xa daily) should be reserved for high risk general surgery and orthopaedic operations. Compression elastic stockings and intermittent pneumatic compression may protect high risk patients when used with anticoagulants. They are also effective when used alone in moderate risk patients where anticoagulants are contraindicated.

### Orthopaedic surgery

In very high risk patients, such as those undergoing major orthopaedic operations, high dose low molecular weight heparin or warfarin is appropriate. The current recommended length of anticoagulant prophylaxis is 7-10 days with low molecular weight heparin or warfarin. Extended use may provide additional benefit. Routine screening with duplex ultrasonography is not helpful. Hirudin seems to be superior to low molecular weight heparin and low dose unfractionated

### Clinical probability for pulmonary embolism

| Clinical feature | Score |
|---|---|
| Deep vein thrombosis suspected: | |
|    Clinical features of deep vein thrombosis | 3.0 |
|    Recent prolonged immobility or surgery | 1.5 |
|    Active cancer | 1.0 |
|    History of deep vein thrombosis or pulmonary embolism | 1.5 |
| Haemoptysis | 1.0 |
| Resting heart rate > 100 beats/min | 1.5 |
| No alternative explanation for acute breathlessness or pleuritic chest pain | 3.0 |

>6 = high probability (60%); 2-6 = moderate probability (20%); <1.5 = low probability (3-4%)

### Thromboembolic risk stratification for surgery patients

- *Low risk*—Uncomplicated surgery in patients aged <40 years with minimal immobility postoperatively and no risk factors
- *Moderate risk*—Any surgery in patients aged 40-60 years, major surgery in patients <40 years and no other risk factors, minor surgery in patients with one or more risk factors
- *High risk*—Major surgery in patients aged >60 years, major surgery in patients aged 40-60 years with one or more risk factors
- *Very high risk*—Major surgery in patients aged >40 years with previous venous thromboembolism, cancer or known hypercoagulable state, major orthopaedic surgery, elective neurosurgery, multiple trauma, or acute spinal cord injury

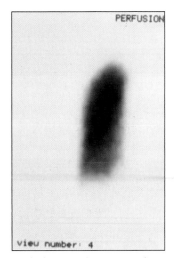 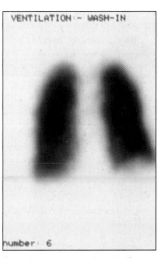

Ventilation-perfusion scan showing massive pulmonary thromboembolism, showing a mismatch between (left) perfusion and (right) ventilation scans

### Key points

- Understanding Virchow's triad aids the treatment of venous thromboembolism
- Numerous situations and risk factors can contribute to venous thromboembolism
- Diagnosis of venous thromboembolism depends upon a combination of history, risk factors, and investigations
- Antithrombotic prophylaxis is safe and effective

heparin as prophylaxis in patients undergoing elective hip replacements but is still not universally available.

## Neurosurgery, multiple traumas, and spinal cord injuries

Intermittent pneumatic compression is the prophylaxis of choice for elective neurosurgery. Among the low molecular weight heparins, only enoxaparin 30 mg twice daily has been shown to reduce venous thromboembolism without excess bleeding after elective neurosurgery, multiple traumas, or spinal cord injuries and so may be used in these situations. Other low molecular weight heparins have either not been tested or have not conclusively been shown to be of benefit in this setting.

## Medical conditions

In general medical patients including heart failure and respiratory failure, both unfractionated heparin and low molecular weight heparin have been shown to be effective in reducing the risk of venous thromboembolism. Low molecular weight heparin has been shown to be more effective than heparin in stroke. Low dose heparin has been shown to be effective in acute myocardial infarction but this is now largely historic because myocardial infarction patients receive therapeutic dose anticoagulants.

## Other considerations

Combined approaches using drugs and physical methods may be better at preventing thromboembolism than physical methods alone. However, compression elastic stockings and intermittent pneumatic compression may be used for moderate or high risk patients when anticoagulation is contraindicated or best avoided. Inferior vena cava filter placement should be reserved for patients at very high risk of venous thromboembolism where anticoagulation as well as physical methods are contraindicated. Inferior vena cava filter placement tends to cause a long term increase of recurrent deep vein thrombosis, even though the immediate risk of postoperative pulmonary embolism is reduced.

## Further reading

- Haemostasis and Thrombosis Task Force of the British Society for Haematology. Guidelines on anticoagulation: third edition. *Br J Haematol* 1998;101:374-87
- Hyers TM, Agnelli G, Hull RD, Morris TA, Samama M, Tapson V, et al. Antithrombotic therapy for venous thromboembolic disease. *Chest* 2001;119:176-93S
- Kearon C, Hirsh J. Management of anticoagulation before and after elective surgery. *N Engl J Med* 1997;336:1506-11
- Simonneau G, Sors H, Charbonnier B, Page Y, Labaan JP, Azarian R et al. A comparison of low molecular weight heparin with unfractionated heparin for acute pulmonary embolism. *N Engl J Med* 1997;337;663-9
- Turpie AG, Bauer KA, Eriksson BI, Lassen MR. Fondaparinus vs enoxaparin for the prevention of venous thromboembolism in major orthopedic surgery: a meta-analysis of 4 randomised double blind studies. *Arch Intern Med* 2002;162:1833-40
- Walker ID, Greaves M, Preston FE. Guideline: Investigation and management of heritable thrombophilia. *Br J Haematol* 2001:114;512-28

## Evidence based use of antithrombotic prophylaxis

### General surgery
- *Low risk*— Early mobilisation
- *Moderate risk*—UH 5000 IU 12 hourly starting two hours before surgery, or low molecular weight heparin <3400 anti-Xa IU daily*, or compression elastic stockings, or intermittent pneumatic compression
- *High risk*—Low molecular weight heparin >3400 anti-Xa IU daily† plus compression elastic stockings, or unfractionated heparin 5000 IU eight hourly starting two hours before surgery plus compression elastic stockings, or intermittent pneumatic compression if anticoagulation contraindicated
- *Very high risk*—Perioperative warfarin (INR 2-3), low molecular weight heparin >3400 anti-Xa IU daily† plus compression elastic stockings, or prolonged low molecular weight heparin therapy plus compression elastic stockings

### Major orthopaedic surgery
- *Elective hip replacement*—Recombinant hirudin 15 mg twice daily, unfractionated heparin 3500 IU eight hourly with postoperative adjustments (APTT 1.2-1.5), or low molecular weight heparin >3400 anti-Xa IU daily†, or perioperative warfarin (INR 2-3), or fondaparinux 2.5 mg daily
- *Elective knee replacement*—Low molecular weight heparin >3400 anti-Xa IU daily†, or perioperative warfarin (INR 2-3), or fondaparinux 2.5 mg daily, intermittent pneumatic compression
- *Surgery for hip fracture*—Low molecular weight heparin >3400 anti-Xa IU daily†, or perioperative warfarin (INR 2-3), or fondaparinux 2.5 mg daily

### Elective neurosurgery
- Intermittent pneumatic compression, enoxaparin 30 mg twice daily

### Acute spinal cord injury
- Enoxaparin 30 mg twice daily

### Trauma
- Enoxaparin 30 mg twice daily

### Acute myocardial infarction
- Low dose unfractionated heparin 5000 IU twice daily, full dose unfractionated heparin 40 000 IU infusion over 24 hours, elastic stockings, and early mobilisation

### Ischaemic stroke
- Low dose unfractionated heparin 5000 IU twice daily

### Other medical conditions including congestive heart failure
- Enoxaparin 40 mg once daily or 30 U twice daily, dalteparin 2500 IU daily, low dose unfractionated heparin 5000 IU twice daily

### Cancer patients receiving chemotherapy
- Low dose warfarin (INR <2), dalteparin 2500 IU daily

*Dalteparin 2500 IU once daily starting two hours before surgery
Enoxaparin 20 mg once daily starting two hours before surgery
Nadroparin 3100 IU once daily starting two hours before surgery
Tinzaparin 3500 IU once daily starting two hours before surgery
†Dalteparin 5000 IU once daily starting 10-12 hours before surgery
Danaparoid 750 IU twice daily starting one to two hours before surgery
Enoxaparin 40 mg once daily starting 10-12 hours before surgery or 30 mg twice daily starting after surgery
Tinzaparin 50 IU/kg once daily starting two hours before surgery

The box showing evidence based use of antithrombotic prophylaxis is adapted from the 6th ACCP guidelines Geerts WH, et al. *Chest* 2001;119:132-75S. The figure showing Plasma D-dimer concentrations on day of presentation according to final diagnosis is adapted from Bounameaux H, et al. *Lancet* 1991;337:196-200.

# 4  Venous thromboembolism: treatment strategies

Alexander G G Turpie, Bernard S P Chin, Gregory Y H Lip

Pulmonary embolism and deep vein thrombosis are treated using similar drugs and physical methods. The efficacy of intravenous infusion of unfractionated heparin was first proved in a randomised trial in 1960. Subsequently, trials concentrated on the dose, duration of infusion, mode of administration, and combination with warfarin treatment. Later trials have reported the efficacy and cost effectiveness of low molecular weight heparin compared with unfractionated heparin.

## Unfractionated heparin

Unfractionated heparin, administered by continuous infusion or subcutaneous injections adjusted to achieve activated partial thromboplastin time (APTT) greater than 1.5, is effective as initial treatment of venous thromboembolism. Initial heparinisation should be followed by long term anticoagulation with oral anticoagulants. APTT is a global coagulation test and not specific for heparin, and it is also influenced by various plasma proteins and clotting factors. Measuring plasma heparin levels is more accurate but it is impractical and expensive. A sensible approach is to standardise the APTT with plasma heparin within each laboratory.

The most common mistake when starting heparin treatment is failure to achieve adequate anticoagulation. APTT ratios of less than 1.5 during the first few days of heparin therapy increase the long term risk of venous thromboembolism recurrence. Hence, the initial bolus dose should be adequate and APTT monitored every six hours during the first 24 hours of heparin infusion.

Oral anticoagulants may be started at the same time and should be continued for at least three to six months, depending on the individual. The optimal duration of intravenous heparin treatment is five to seven days because this is the time needed to obtain an adequate and persistent reduction in the vitamin K dependent clotting factors with oral anticoagulants such as warfarin. Heparin can then be stopped when concomitant use with warfarin has achieved an international normalised ratio (INR) of 2-3 for at least 48 hours. In patients with large ileofemoral vein thromboses or major pulmonary embolism, heparin infusion can be continued for up to 10 days.

Heparin use for more than five to six days is associated with a rare risk of thrombocytopenia. In a recent trial, only one of 308 patients (0.32%) who received unfractionated heparin for acute pulmonary embolism developed a thrombocytopenia, whereas none of 304 patients receiving low molecular weight heparin had this problem. The thrombocytopenia is normally mild, but precipitous falls in platelet count to less than $100 \times 10^9/l$ can occur. When this happens, antibody mediated injury to platelets should be suspected. As this condition may be associated with arterial or venous thromboembolism, heparin should be stopped and warfarin use delayed. Alternative anticoagulation cover should be given by danaparoid, a heparinoid, or hirudin, a thrombin inhibitor, until the platelet count rises above 100 000 and it is safe to start warfarin. Unfractionated heparin has also been reported to increase platelet activation in vivo: low molecular weight heparin had no such effect.

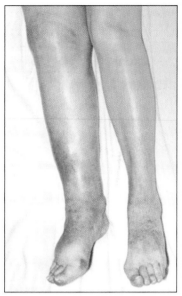

Right ileofemoral deep vein thrombosis

**Antithrombotic treatment is often inadequate in the first few days, predisposing to recurrences. Anticoagulation with warfarin after discharge should continue for at least three months, possibly six months. Low molecular weight heparin is as efficacious as unfractionated heparin in prophylaxis and treatment**

---

**Initial antithrombotic therapy for deep vein thrombosis with unfractionated heparin**

1  Check baseline APTT, prothrombin time, full blood count
2  Confirm there are no contraindications to heparin therapy
3  Intravenous bolus 5000 IU
4  Choose between:
   *Continuous unfractionated heparin infusion*—Start infusion at 18 IU/kg/hour (~30 000/24 hours in a 70 kg man)
   Check APTT every six hours for first 24 hours, then daily thereafter
   Aim for APTT 1.5-2.5 × normal
   Recheck APTT at six hours after each adjustment
   Continue infusion for five to seven days
   *Subcutaneous*—Start at 17 500 IU every 12 hours (or 250 IU/kg every 12 hours)
5  Check platelet count daily for thrombocytopenia
6  Warfarin therapy can be started on the first day of heparin therapy according to local protocol
7  Continue heparin for at least four to five days after starting warfarin
8  Stop heparin when INR greater than 2 for more than 48 hours
9  Continue warfarin therapy for at least three months keeping INR between 2 and 3 (target 2.5)

---

# Low molecular weight heparin

Low molecular weight heparin has a more predictable relation between dose and response than unfractionated heparin and does not need monitoring or adjustments if the dose is based on patient body weight. Low molecular weight heparin is also associated with lower risk of thrombocytopenia. Its use in deep vein thrombosis and pulmonary embolism is now firmly established: many trials and meta-analysis have confirmed its superior efficacy, safer profile, and greater cost effectiveness over unfractionated heparins. However, all low molecular weight heparins are different, and trials for one product cannot be extrapolated to another. The introduction of low molecular weight heparin has advanced antithrombotic therapy by providing effective anticoagulation without the need for monitoring or adjustments. It also allows patients with uncomplicated deep vein thrombosis to be treated in the community, saving an average of four to five days' admission per patient.

# Coumarins

Warfarin is the most widely used oral anticoagulant for treating venous thromboembolism. It is well absorbed from the gut, metabolised in the liver, and excreted in urine. The lag time for warfarin to take effect may be related to the natural clearance of normal clotting factors from plasma. Of the vitamin K dependent clotting factors, factor II takes the longest to clear. Warfarin monitoring is performed using an INR rather than prothrombin time, which may vary between laboratories. Warfarin interacts with many other drugs and alcohol. It is also teratogenic and may induce spontaneous abortion.

A target INR range of 2-3 is standard for treatment of venous thromboembolism. Higher levels tend to increase incidence of bleeding without reducing recurrent thromboembolism and so are unnecessary. The exception to this is for patients with the antiphospholipid antibody syndrome, where the risk of recurrent venous thromboembolism is high. Here, an INR of 3-4.5 is recommended. Warfarin should be started in conjunction with heparin or low molecular weight heparin when the diagnosis of venous thromboembolism is confirmed, although local protocols may vary in their starting doses and titration schedule. As indicated, heparin should be continued concomitantly for five days and until INR is >2.

Warfarin therapy should then be maintained for at least three months in all patients. However, it has recently been established that longer treatments (such as six months) may be necessary. Patients without a readily identifiable risk factor (idiopathic venous thromboembolism) have higher rates of recurrences. These recurrences can be reduced by prolonged anticoagulation. However, there is a corresponding rise in bleeding complications with prolonged anticoagulation. Current recommendations advocate anticoagulation for at least six months for the first presentation of idiopathic venous thromboembolism. Patients with recurrent venous thromboembolism and hypercoagulable states (acquired or inherited) or with cancer (especially while receiving chemotherapy) should take anticoagulation therapy for at least a year, and perhaps indefinitely.

# Thrombolytic therapy

Unlike heparin and warfarin, which prevent extension and recurrences of thrombosis, thrombolytic agents (including streptokinase, urokinase, and tissue plasminogen activator) lyse the thrombi. It is therefore unsurprising that patients with

**Advantages of low molecular weight heparin over unfractionated heparin**

- More reliable relation between dose and response
- Does not need monitoring
- Does not need dose adjustments
- Lower incidence of thrombocytopenia
- No excess bleeding
- Can be administered by patient at home
- Saves about five to six days' admission per patient

**Duration of anticoagulation therapy for venous thromboembolism***

**Three to six months**
- First event with reversible† or time limited risk factor (patient may have underlying factor V Leiden or prothrombin 20210 mutation)

**More than six months**
- Idiopathic venous thromboembolism, first event

**A year to life time**
- First event‡ with cancer (until resolved), anticardiolipin antibody, antithrombin deficiency
- Recurrent event, idiopathic or with thrombophilia

*All recommendations are subject to modification by individual characteristics including patient preference, age, comorbidity, and likelihood of recurrence
†Reversible or time limited risk factors such as surgery, trauma, immobilisation, and oestrogen use
‡Proper duration of therapy is unclear in first event with homozygous factor V Leiden, homocystinaemia, deficiency of protein C or S, or multiple thrombophilias; and in recurrent events with reversible risk factors

**Recent trials with the oral thrombin inhibitor, ximelagatran suggest that, in certain circumstances, this agent may be an alternative to warfarin for the management of venous thromboembolism, without the need for anticoagulation monitoring**

**Thrombolytic regimens for pulmonary embolism**

1 Check suitability of patient for thrombolysis
2 Choose between:
 *Streptokinase*—250 000 IU loading dose then 100 000 IU/hour for 24 hours
 *Urokinase*—4400 IU/kg loading dose then 2200 IU/kg/hour for 12 hours
 *Alteplase*—100 mg intravenously over an hour
3 Check APTT two to four hours after starting infusion: >10 seconds prolongation indicates active fibrinolysis
4 Start heparin at 5000-10 000 IU loading followed by 15-25 units/kg/hour when APTT < 2
5 Adjust according to local protocol to keep APTT 1.5-2.5

pulmonary embolism treated with streptokinase and urokinase are three times more likely to show clot resolution than patients taking heparin alone. Even so, thrombolytic therapy of pulmonary embolism does not dissolve the clot completely as it does with acute coronary thrombosis, and increases the risk of bleeding. Occasionally, thrombolytic therapy is administered via a catheter placed in the pulmonary artery. The catheter can be used to "disrupt" the thrombus before starting the drug.

Until there is more evidence that thrombolytic therapy reduces mortality in pulmonary embolism, this treatment should be reserved for patients with massive pulmonary embolism, cardiorespiratory compromise, and low risk of bleeding. Evidence is emerging that streptokinase can decrease swelling and pain in deep vein thrombosis. Again, further trials are needed before this can be recommended routinely.

## Physical methods

Non-drug treatments include physically preventing embolisation of the thrombi and extraction of thromboemboli (usually from the pulmonary vasculature).

Inferior vena cava filters may be used when anticoagulation is contraindicated in patients at high risk of proximal deep vein thrombosis extension or embolisation. The filter is normally inserted via the internal jugular or femoral vein. It is then advanced under fluoroscopic guidance to the inferior vena cava. Filters are now available that are easy to insert, and complications are low in skilled hands. For now, this technique should be considered in patients with recurrent symptomatic pulmonary embolism and as primary prophylaxis of thromboembolism in patients at high risk of bleeding (such as patients with extensive trauma or visceral cancer), although the evidence is based on uncontrolled case series. The only randomised trial showed a reduction in pulmonary embolism but no improvement in short or long term survival, because of greater risk of recurrent deep vein thrombosis in patients who received a filter.

Other mechanical and surgical treatments are usually reserved for massive pulmonary embolism where drug treatments have failed or are contraindicated. None of these methods has shown a long term reduction in mortality, but better techniques have led to acceptable complication rates and warrant further evaluation.

## Treatment during pregnancy

Unfractionated heparin and low molecular weight heparin do not cross the placenta and are probably safe for the fetus during pregnancy. Oral anticoagulants cross the placenta and can cause fetal bleeding and malformations. Pregnant women with venous thromboembolism can be treated with therapeutic doses of subcutaneous heparin or low molecular weight heparin until after delivery, when warfarin can be used safely. These issues are developed in chapter 14.

The data on duration of anticoagulation therapy for venous thromboembolism is adapted from the 6th ACCP guidelines Hyers TM, et al. Antithrombotic therapy for venous thromboembolic disease. *Chest* 2001;119:176-93S

---

**Indications for inferior vena cava filter placement**

- Patients at high risk of proximal deep vein thrombosis extension where anticoagulation is contraindicated
- Recurrent venous thromboembolism despite adequate anticoagulation
- Chronic recurrent venous thromboembolism with pulmonary hypertension
- Simultaneous surgical pulmonary embolectomy or endarterectomy

---

**Mechanical and surgical treatment of pulmonary embolism**

- Inferior vena cava filter placement
  *Indications*—See box above
- Pulmonary embolectomy
  *Indication*—Massive pulmonary embolism compromising cardiac output where thrombolysis has failed or is contraindicated
  Experienced cardiac surgical cover essential
  Where available, catheter transvenous extraction of emboli may be an alternative to pulmonary embolectomy
- Pulmonary endarterectomy
  *Indication*—Chronic recurrent pulmonary embolism with secondary pulmonary hypertension

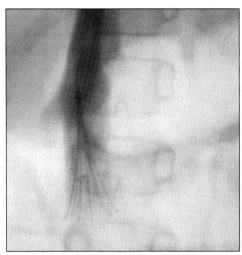

Vena cavagram showing umbrella delivery device for filter inserted into the inferior vena cava through the jugular vein

---

**Further reading**

- Decousus H, Leizorovicz A, Parent F, Page Y, Tardy B, Girard P, et al. A clinical trial of vena caval filters in the prevention of pulmonary embolism in patients with proximal deep vein thrombosis. *N Engl J Med* 1998;338:409-15
- Geerts WH, Heit JA, Clagett GP, Pineo GF, Colwell CW, Anderson FA Jr, et al. Prevention of venous thromboembolism. *Chest* 2000;119:132-75S
- Heit JA, O'Fallon WM, Petterson T, Lohse CM, Silverstein MD, Mohr DN, et al. Relative impact of risk factors for deep vein thrombosis and pulmonary embolism. *Arch Intern Med* 2002;162:1245-8
- Levine M, Gent M, Hirsch J, Leclerc J, Anderson D, Weitz J, et al. A comparison of low-molecular-weight heparin administered primarily at home with unfractionated heparin administered in the hospital for proximal deep-vein thrombosis. *N Engl J Med* 1996;334:677-81
- Walker ID, Greaves M, Preston FE. Guideline: investigation and management of heritable thrombophilia. *Br J Haematol* 2001;114:512-28

# 5 Antithrombotic therapy for atrial fibrillation: clinical aspects

Gregory Y H Lip, Robert G Hart, Dwayne S G Conway

Atrial fibrillation is the commonest sustained disorder of cardiac rhythm. Although patients often present with symptoms caused by haemodynamic disturbance associated with the rhythm itself, the condition carries an increased risk of arterial thromboembolism and ischaemic stroke due to embolisation of thrombi that form within the left atrium of the heart. Presence of the arrhythmia confers about a fivefold increase in stroke risk, an absolute risk of about 4.5% a year, although the precise annual stroke risk ranges from <1% to >12%, according to the presence or absence of certain clinical and echocardiographically identifiable risk factors.

From trial data, patients with paroxysmal atrial fibrillation seem to carry the same risk as those with persistent atrial fibrillation. The same criteria can be used to identify high risk patients, although it is unclear whether the risk is dependent on the frequency and duration of the paroxysms.

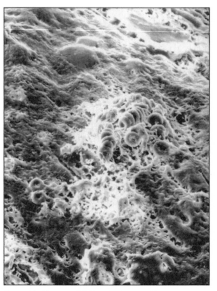

Severely damaged left atrial appendage endocardial surface with thrombotic mass in a patient with atrial fibrillation and mitral valve disease

## Evidence from clinical trials

It is well established that antithrombotic therapy confers thromboprophylaxis in patients with atrial fibrillation who are at risk of thromboembolism. A recent meta-analysis of antithrombotic therapy in atrial fibrillation showed that adjusted dose warfarin reduced stroke by about 60%, with absolute risk reductions of 3% a year for primary prevention and 8% a year for secondary prevention (numbers needed to treat for one year to prevent one stroke of 33 and 13, respectively). In contrast, aspirin reduced stroke by about 20%, with absolute risk reductions of 1.5% a year for primary prevention and 2.5% a year for secondary prevention (numbers needed to treat of 66 and 40, respectively). Relative to aspirin, adjusted dose warfarin reduced the risk by about 40%, and the relative risk reduction was similar for primary and secondary prevention, and for disabling and non-disabling strokes. However, these data, obtained from well planned clinical trials recruiting patients with relatively stable conditions, are unlikely to be fully extrapolable to all patients in general practice, so that some caution is advised.

Overall, warfarin (generally at a dose to maintain an international normalised ratio (INR) of 2-3) is significantly more effective than aspirin in treating atrial fibrillation in patients at high risk of stroke, especially in preventing disabling cardioembolic strokes. The effect of aspirin seems to be on the smaller, non-cardioembolic strokes from which elderly, and often hypertensive, patients with atrial fibrillation are not spared.

Recent clinical trials have suggested that there is no role for minidose warfarin (1 mg/day regardless of INR), alone or in combination with antiplatelet agents or aspirin, as thromboprophylaxis in atrial fibrillation. However, the role of other antiplatelet agents (such as indobufen and dipyridamole) in atrial fibrillation is still unclear. One small trial (SIFA) compared treatment with indobufen, a reversible cyclo-oxygenase inhibitor, with full dose warfarin for secondary prevention and found no statistical difference between the two groups, who were well matched for confounding risk factors. Trials of other antiplatelet and antithrombotic drugs (including low molecular weight heparin) have been performed but have generally been too small and underpowered to show significant differences. Large

> **Randomised controlled trials have shown the benefit of warfarin and, to a lesser extent, aspirin in reducing the incidence of stroke in patients with atrial fibrillation without greatly increasing the risk of haemorrhagic stroke and extracranial haemorrhage. However, anticoagulant therapy is still underprescribed in patients with atrial fibrillation, particularly in elderly patients, who stand to benefit most**

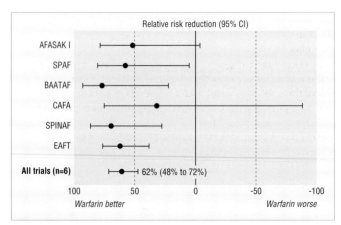

Meta-analysis of trials comparing warfarin with placebo in reducing the risk of thromboembolism in patients with atrial fibrillation
AFASAK=Copenhagen atrial fibrillation, aspirin, and anticoagulation study; BAATAF=Boston area anticoagulation trial for atrial fibrillation; CAFA=Canadian atrial fibrillation anticoagulation study; EAFT=European atrial fibrillation trial; SPAF=Stroke prevention in atrial fibrillation study; SPINAF=Stroke prevention in non-rheumatic atrial fibrillation

multinational trials comparing a direct thrombin inhibitor (ximelagatran) with adjusted dose warfarin in over 7000 patients with atrial fibrillation at high risk of stroke and thromboembolism suggest that this agent may be an alternative to warfarin, without the need for anticoagulation monitoring.

The reduction in relative risk with warfarin applies equally to primary and secondary prevention but, as history of stroke confers an increased annual stroke risk (12% v 4.5%), the absolute risk reduction is greater for secondary prevention. The number of patients with atrial fibrillation needing treatment with warfarin to prevent one stroke is therefore about three times greater in primary prevention (37) than in secondary prevention (12).

Treatment with full dose anticoagulation carries the potential risk of major bleeding, including intracranial haemorrhage. Meta-analysis of the initial five primary prevention trials plus a further secondary prevention trial suggests the risk of haemorrhagic stroke is only marginally increased from 0.1% to 0.3% a year. Higher rates of major haemorrhage were seen in elderly patients and those with higher intensity anticoagulation. Further recent trials have confirmed an increased bleeding risk in patients with INR >3.

## Antiplatelet therapy in atrial fibrillation

Several clinical trials have studied the effects of aspirin in atrial fibrillation, with doses ranging from 25 mg twice daily to 1200 mg a day. Overall, aspirin reduces the relative risk of stroke by about 20% (a figure which just reaches statistical significance) with no apparent benefit of increasing aspirin dose. Aspirin seems to carry greater benefit in reducing smaller non-disabling strokes than disabling strokes. This may be due to an effect primarily on carotid and cerebral artery platelet thrombus formation, rather than on formation of intra-atrial thrombus. A meta-analysis of trials directly comparing full dose warfarin with aspirin confirmed significant reductions in stroke risk about three times greater with warfarin. The SPAF III trial demonstrates that addition of fixed low doses of warfarin to aspirin treatment is not sufficient to achieve the benefits of full dose warfarin alone.

## Putting the evidence into practice

Despite the evidence from the trials, many doctors are reluctant to start warfarin treatment for patients with atrial fibrillation. This could be due to fears (of patient and doctor) of haemorrhagic complications in an elderly population, logistical problems of INR monitoring, and a lack of consensus guidelines on which patients to treat and the ideal target INR. Such attitudes may result in otherwise avoidable stroke and arterial thromboembolism. A systematic evidence based approach needs to be encouraged, targeting appropriate antithrombotic therapy at those patients who stand to gain most benefit (those at greatest risk of thromboembolism) and using levels of anticoagulation that have been proved both effective and reasonably safe for both primary and secondary prevention of stroke, if we are to realise in clinical practice the large reduction in incidence of stroke achieved in the clinical trials.

# Who to treat?

Even though there are impressive figures for relative risk reduction with warfarin, the figures for absolute risk reduction (more important in clinical practice) depend greatly on the underlying risk of stroke if untreated. Elderly patients are often denied anticoagulant therapy because of fears of increased haemorrhage risk. However, the benefits of anticoagulant therapy are greater for elderly patients because of the increased

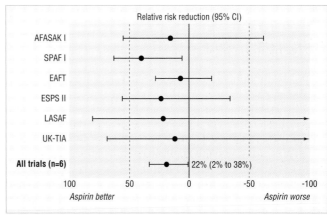

Meta-analysis of trials comparing aspirin with placebo in reducing risk of thromboembolism in patients with atrial fibrillation
AFASAK=Copenhagen atrial fibrillation, aspirin, and anticoagulation study; EAFT=European atrial fibrillation trial; ESPS II= European stroke prevention study II; LASAF=Low-dose aspirin, stroke, and atrial fibrillation pilot study; SPAF=Stroke prevention in atrial fibrillation study; UK-TIA=United Kingdom TIA study

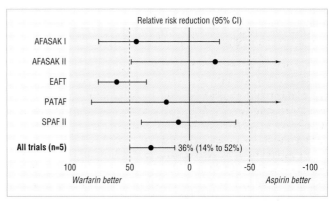

Meta-analysis of trials comparing warfarin with aspirin in reducing risk of thromboembolism in patients with atrial fibrillation
AFASAK=Copenhagen atrial fibrillation, aspirin, and anticoagulation study; EAFT=European atrial fibrillation trial; PATAF=Prevention of arterial thromboembolism in atrial fibrillation; SPAF=Stroke prevention in atrial fibrillation study

## Independent predictors of ischaemic stroke in non-valve atrial fibrillation

**Consistent predictors**
- Old age
- Hypertension
- Previous stroke or transient ischaemic attack
- Left ventricular dysfunction*

**Inconsistent predictors**
- Diabetes
- Systolic blood pressure >160 mm Hg†
- Women, especially older than 75 years
- Postmenopausal hormone replacement therapy
- Coronary artery disease

**Factors which decrease the risk of stroke**
- Moderate to severe mitral regurgitation
- Regular alcohol use (>14 drinks in two weeks)

*Recent clinical congestive cardiac failure or moderate to severe systolic dysfunction on echocardiography
†In some analyses, systolic blood pressure >160 mm Hg remained an independent predictor after adjustment for hypertension

# ABC of Antithrombotic Therapy

underlying thromboembolic risk. Conversely, young patients at relatively low risk of stroke have less to gain from full dose anticoagulation as there may be little difference between the number of strokes prevented and the number of haemorrhagic complications. Risk stratification is possible using the clinical and echocardiographic parameters and can be used to target treatment at the most appropriate patients.

Risk stratification for thromboprophylaxis can be undertaken in many ways. Clinical risk factors would assist with risk stratification in most cases. Although echocardiography is not mandatory, it would help refine risk stratification in cases of uncertainty. Based on echocardiographic data on 1066 patients, the Atrial Fibrillation Investigators reported that the only independent predictor of stroke risk was moderate or severe left ventricular dysfunction on two dimensional echocardiography. Left atrial size on M mode echocardiography was not an independent predictor on multivariate analysis. Transoesophageal echocardiography is rarely needed to undertake risk stratification, but "high risk" features include the presence of dense spontaneous echocardiographic contrast

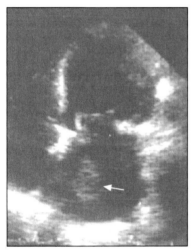

Two dimensional echocardiography showing left atrial thrombus in patient with prosthetic valve

## Practical guidelines for antithrombotic therapy in non-valvar atrial fibrillation

### Assess risk, and reassess regularly

**High risk (annual risk of cerebrovascular accident=8-12%)**
- All patients with previous transient ischaemic attack or cerebrovascular accident
- All patients aged ≥75 with diabetes or hypertension
- All patients with clinical evidence of valve disease, heart failure, thyroid disease, and impaired left ventricular function on echocardiography*

*Treatment*—Give warfarin (target INR 2-3) if no contraindications and possible in practice

**Moderate risk (annual risk of cerebrovascular accident=4%)**
- All patients <65 with clinical risk factors: diabetes, hypertension, peripheral vascular disease, ischaemic heart disease
- All patients >65 not in high risk group

*Treatment*—Either warfarin (INR 2-3) or aspirin 75-300 mg daily. In view of insufficient clear cut evidence, treatment may be decided on individual cases. Referral and echocardiography may help

**Low risk (annual risk=1%)**
- All patients aged <65 with no history of embolism, hypertension, diabetes, or other clinical risk factors

*Treatment*—Give aspirin 75-300 mg daily

*Echocardiogram not needed for routine risk assessment but refines clinical risk stratification in case of moderate or severe left ventricular dysfunction (see figure below) and valve disease. A large atrium per se is not an independent risk factor on multivariate analysis

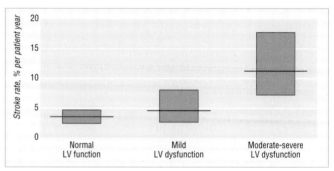

Effect of left ventricular funtion on stroke rate in atrial fibrillation
LV=left ventricle

---

## Different risk stratification schemes for primary prevention of stroke in non-valvar atrial fibrillation

| Study | Risk | | |
|---|---|---|---|
| | **High** | **Intermediate** | **Low** |
| Atrial Fibrillation Investigators (1994) | High to intermediate risk: Age >65 years, History of hypertension, Diabetes | | Age <65 years, No high risk features |
| American College of Chest Physicians Consensus (1998) | Age >75 years, History of hypertension, Left ventricular dysfunction†, >1 moderate risk factor | Age 65-75 years, Diabetes, Coronary disease (thyrotoxicosis)* | Age <65 years, No risk factors |
| Stroke Prevention in Atrial Fibrillation | Women aged ≥75 years, Systolic blood pressure >160 mm Hg, Left ventricular dysfunction‡ | History of hypertension, No high risk features | No high risk features, No history of hypertension |
| Lip (1999) | Patients aged >75 years and with diabetes or hypertension, Patients with clinical evidence of heart failure, thyroid disease, and impaired left ventricular function on echocardiography§ | Patients aged <65 years with clinical risk factors: diabetes, hypertension, peripheral arterial disease, ischaemic heart disease, Patients aged >65 not in high risk group | Patients aged <65 years with no risk factors |

*Patients with thyrotoxicosis were excluded from participation in the test cohort
†Moderate to severe left ventricular dysfunction on echocardiography
‡Recent congestive heart failure or fractional shortening ≤25% by M mode echocardiography
§Echocardiography not needed for routine risk assessment but refines clinical risk stratification in case of impaired left ventricular function and valve disease

(often with low atrial appendage velocities, indicating stasis), the presence of thrombus of the atrial appendage, and complex aortic plaque.

## Which INR range?

The evidence suggests that INR levels greater than 3 may result in an excess rate of haemorrhage, whereas low dose warfarin regimens (with INR maintained below 1.5) do not achieve the reductions in stroke of higher doses. An INR range of between 2 and 3 has been shown to be highly effective without leading to excessive haemorrhage and should therefore be recommended for all patients with atrial fibrillation treated with warfarin unless they have another indication for higher levels of anticoagulation (such as a mechanical heart valve). Although INR monitoring is often coordinated by hospital based anticoagulant clinics, general practitioners are likely to play a more important part with the development of near patient INR testing.

Particular care must be taken and INR levels closely monitored when warfarin is used in elderly patients. It has been suggested that an INR of between 1.6 and 2.5 can provide substantial, albeit partial, efficacy (estimated to be nearly 90% of the highest intensities). Given the uncertainty about the safety of INRs >2.5 for atrial fibrillation patients over 75 years, a target INR of 2 (range 1.6-2.5) may be a reasonable compromise between an increased risk of haemorrhage and a reduced risk of thrombotic stroke for some patients within this age group, in the absence of additional risk factors, pending further data about the safety of higher intensities.

The ongoing MRC sponsored Birmingham atrial fibrillation trial of anticoagulation in the aged (BAFTA) is comparing warfarin with aspirin in atrial fibrillation patients over 75 years to further define the relative benefits and risks.

## DC cardioversion

No hard evidence exists in the literature that restoration of sinus rhythm by whatever means reduces stroke risk. Transoesophageal echocardiography performed immediately before cardioversion (to exclude intra-atrial thrombus) may allow DC cardioversion to be performed without prior anticoagulation. However, as the thromboembolic risk may persist for a few weeks postprocedure, it is still recommended that patients receive warfarin for at least four weeks afterwards.

The figures showing a severely damaged left atrial appendage endocardial surface is reproduced from Goldsmith I et al, *Am Heart J* 2000;140:777-84 with permission from Mosby Inc. The figures showing results of trials comparing warfarin with placebo, aspirin with placebo, and warfarin with aspirin are adapted from Hart RG et al, *Ann Intern Med* 1999;131:492-501. The independent predictors of ischaemic stroke are adapted from Hart RG et al, *Ann Intern Med* 1999;131:688-95. The practical guidelines for antithrombotic therapy in non-valvar patients is adapted from Lip GYH, *Lancet* 1999;353:4-6. The table containing risk stratification schemes for primary prevention of stroke is adapted from Pearce LA et al, *Am J Med* 2000;109:45-51. Guidelines for transoesophageal echocardiography guided cardioversion is adapted from the ACUTE Study, *N Engl J Med* 2001;344:1411-20. The recommendations for anticoagulation for cardioversion of atrial fibrillation are based on the 6th ACCP Consensus Conference on Antithrombotic Therapy. Albers GW et al, *Chest* 2001;119:194-206S.

### Recommendations for anticoagulation for cardioversion of atrial fibrillation

- For elective cardioversion of atrial fibrillation of >48 hours duration start warfarin treatment (INR 2-3) three weeks before and continue for four weeks after cardioversion
- In urgent and emergency cardioversion administer intravenous heparin followed by warfarin
- Treat atrial flutter similarly
- No anticoagulation treatment is required for supraventricular tachycardia or atrial fibrillation of <48 hours duration
- Continue anticoagulation in patients with multiple risk factors or those at high risk of recurrent thromboembolism

Based on the 6th ACCP Consensus Conference on Antithrombotic Therapy

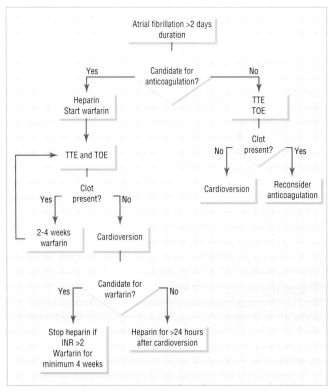

Guidelines for transoesophageal echocardiography guided cardioversion
TOE=transoesophageal echocardiography; TTE=transthoracic echocardiography

### Further reading

- Hart RG, Pearce LA, Rothbart RM, McAnulty JH, Asinger RW, Halperin JL. Stroke with intermittent atrial fibrillation: incidence and predictors during aspirin therapy. Stroke Prevention in Atrial Fibrillation Investigators. *J Am Coll Cardiol* 2000;35:183-7
- Lip GYH. Does atrial fibrillation confer a hypercoagulable state? *Lancet* 1995;346:1313-4
- Lip GYH. Thromboprophylaxis for atrial fibrillation. *Lancet* 1999; 353:4-6
- Lip GYH, Kamath S, Freestone B. Acute atrial fibrillation. *Clinical Evidence* June Issue 7. BMJ Publishing Group. 2002
- Straus SE, Majumdar SR, McAlister FA. New edvidence for stroke prevention: scientific review. *JAMA* 2002;288:1388
- Thomson R, Parkin D, Eccles M, Sudlow M, Robinson A. Decision analysis and guidelines for anticoagulant therapy to prevent stroke in patients with atrial fibrillation. *Lancet* 2000;355:956-62

# 6 Antithrombotic therapy for atrial fibrillation: pathophysiology, acute atrial fibrillation, and cardioversion

Gregory Y H Lip, Robert G Hart, Dwayne S G Conway

## Pathophysiology of thromboembolism in atrial fibrillation

The pathophysiological mechanism for thrombus formation and embolism seems to be abnormalities in blood flow within the fibrillating (and possibly dilated) left atrium. These abnormalities predispose to thrombus formation and arterial embolism, especially in the presence of underlying heart disease. The latter (including valvar heart disease, hypertensive heart disease, and poor left ventricular function) substantially increases the risk for stroke and thromboembolism in patients with atrial fibrillation. For example, the thromboembolic risk of atrial fibrillation is 18 times greater if valvar heart disease is present. In addition, a history of stroke, transient ischaemic attack, or other thromboembolism substantially increases the risk of stroke in atrial fibrillation (by 2.5 times). Hypertension and diabetes are also common risk factors for stroke, increasing the risk of stroke in atrial fibrillation by nearly twofold.

### Anatomical aspects

A left atrial diameter of $\geq 4.0$ cm was previously regarded as the strongest single predictor of increased risk of thromboembolisation, but atrial dilatation rarely occurs in isolation without associated clinical risk factors such as hypertension. Thus, in the most recent analysis from the Atrial Fibrillation Investigators, isolated left atrial dilatation by M mode echocardiography was not independently predictive of stroke and thromboembolism on multivariate analysis. Nevertheless, patients with lone atrial fibrillation (that is, those who have no underlying cause for their arrhythmia), have been shown to have a low risk of stroke and usually have an atrial size < 4.0 cm. Left atrial enlargement has also been associated with the presence of "spontaneous echocontrast" on transoesophageal echocardiography. With scanning electron microscopy, the endocardium of the left atrial appendage shows evidence of damage in mitral valve disease, especially in the presence of atrial fibrillation.

### Mechanical aspects

The loss of atrial systolic function reduces stroke volume, leading to a corresponding reduction in cardiac output and increased atrial stasis. The latter results in increased propensity to thrombus formation. The prevalence of thrombus in the left atrial appendage, detected as an incidental finding during transoesophageal echocardiography, has been reported to be about 10-15% in patients admitted with acute atrial fibrillation and up to 30% in patients with atrial fibrillation and recent stroke.

Indeed, after cardioversion from atrial fibrillation to sinus rhythm, there is risk of thromboembolism of about 7% if anticoagulation is not used, with the highest risk one to two weeks after cardioversion. This may reflect mechanical reasons (embolisation of preformed thrombus), but it is more likely that this increased risk is related to atrial dysfunction after cardioversion ("stunning") and the delay of the return of atrial systolic function, which can be up to three weeks or more after cardioversion.

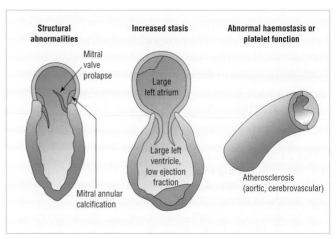

Virchow's triad of thrombogenesis needs the presence of structural abnormalities (for example—atherosclerosis, valve disease), abnormal flow (stasis in left atria, heart failure), and abnormal blood constituents (for example—clotting factors, platelets, etc). All are present in "high risk" patients with atrial fibrillation

**In patients with paroxysmal atrial fibrillation, thromboembolic events seem to cluster in the transition from atrial fibrillation to sinus rhythm, perhaps reflecting embolisation of a preformed clot**

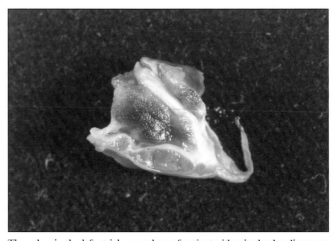

Thrombus in the left atrial appendage of patient with mitral valve disease at surgery

**Atrial fibrillation and hypercoagulability**

It has been recognised for over 150 years that abnormalities in the blood vessel wall, blood flow, and blood constituents (Virchow's triad) may increase the propensity for thrombus formation. Clinical and echocardiographic criteria can help identify the first two of Virchow's postulates for thrombogenesis—namely, abnormalities of blood flow and vessels, such as valvar heart disease and cardiac impairment. Patients with atrial fibrillation also show abnormalities of haemostatic and platelet markers that are unrelated to aetiology and underlying structural heart disease (and alter with antithrombotic therapy and cardioversion), which point towards the presence of a hypercoagulable state in this common arrhythmia. Thus, atrial fibrillation has been described as an arrhythmia which confers a prothrombotic or hypercoaguable state.

# Anticoagulation for atrial fibrillation in special circumstances

**Acute atrial fibrillation**

In patients presenting with de novo atrial fibrillation, a clear history of arrhythmia onset is needed to guide appropriate antithrombotic therapy and timing of cardioversion.

Although no randomised trials have specifically addressed the issue, there is evidence that cardioversion may be safely performed without anticoagulation if the arrhythmia has been present for < 48 hours. However, in one series intra-atrial thrombus was detected by transoesophageal echocardiography in about 15% of patients presenting with acute atrial fibrillation (apparent duration < 48 hours), raising the possibility that the development of intra-atrial thrombus may be faster than previously suspected, or that in many apparent cases of acute atrial fibrillation the arrhythmia developed asymptomatically > 48 hours before. Thus, in cases of uncertainty, anticoagulation is needed. Again, no randomised prospective studies have addressed the use of intravenous unfractionated heparin or subcutaneous low molecular weight heparin derivatives, but both drugs have been used with good results in the acute and pericardioversion periods.

**Atrial fibrillation patients presenting with acute stroke**

The role of antiplatelet drugs after acute stroke in sinus rhythm is well proved, but there is less certainty about the potential benefits and hazards of anticoagulant treatment in patients with atrial fibrillation, particularly the timing of administration. Although the benefits of secondary stroke prevention using warfarin in atrial fibrillation patients are dramatic, it must be certain that there is no ongoing intracerebral haemorrhage (or risk of new intracerebral haemorrhage) before starting the drug.

Previous consensus guidelines from the American College of Chest Physicians state that before any antithrombotic drug is started computed tomography or magnetic resonance imaging scan should be done to confirm the absence of intracranial haemorrhage and to assess the size of any cerebral infarction. In atrial fibrillation patients with no evidence of haemorrhage and small infarct size (or no evidence of infarction) warfarin (INR 2.0-3.0) can be given with minimal risk, provided patients are normotensive. In atrial fibrillation patients with large areas of cerebral infarction, the start of warfarin treatment should be delayed for two weeks because of the potential risk of haemorrhagic transformation. The presence of intracranial haemorrhage is an absolute contraindication to the immediate and future use of anticoagulation for stroke prevention in atrial fibrillation. The mortality benefits of aspirin treatment in acute stroke seen in the international stroke trial and Chinese acute

> The development of intra-atrial thrombus, and thus the immediate risk of thromboembolism, is thought to be temporally related to the duration of the arrhythmia, with minimal risk if the arrhythmia has been present for < 48 hours

**Benefits of anticoagulant treatment in patients with non-rheumatic atrial fibrillation in preventing stroke**

| Stroke risk | NNT (95% CI) to prevent one stroke |
|---|---|
| Low:<br>Age < 65 years, no major risk factors (including previous stroke, systemic embolism, or transient ischaemic attack; hypertension; and poor left ventricular function as determined by a clinical history of heart failure or left ventricular ejection fraction < 50%) | Aspirin 227 (132 to 2500) |
| Low moderate:<br>Age 65-75 years, no major risk factors | Aspirin 152 (88 to 1667)<br>Warfarin 54 (46 to 69) |
| High moderate:<br>Age 65-75 years, no major risk factors but either diabetes or coronary heart disease | Warfarin 32 (28 to 42) |
| High:<br>Age < 75 years with hypertension, left ventricular dysfunction, or both, or age > 75 without other risk factors | Warfarin 14 (12 to 17) |
| Very high:<br>Age > 75 years with hypertension, left ventricular dysfunction, or both, or any age and previous stroke, transient ischaemic attack, or systemic embolism | Warfarin 8 (7 to 10) |

NNT = number needed to treat

stroke trial were less marked in patients with atrial fibrillation, presumably because of the presence of preformed intra-atrial thrombus rather than new localised platelet thrombus adhering to carotid and cerebral artery atheroma.

## Cardioversion of persistent atrial fibrillation

Although there are no randomised studies to show that successful cardioversion of atrial fibrillation reduces the number of subsequent thromboembolic events, the improvement in haemodynamic function and observed reduction in indices of clotting suggest that this may be the case. However, cardioversion is known to increase the short term risk of thromboembolism, and thus, unless the arrhythmia has been present for less than 48 hours, thromboprophylactic measures are needed. The mechanism behind pericardioversion thromboembolism is complex and not entirely understood, but it is likely to be associated with the return of atrial systole, temporary "stunning" of the left atrium before return of systolic function, and possibly an increase in thrombotic tendency caused by the procedure itself. The increase in thromboembolic risk may therefore persist for two weeks or more after successful cardioversion.

The American College of Chest Physicians (ACCP) sixth recommendations for pericardioversion anticoagulation have been summarised in the previous chapter. However, the recent ACUTE study found that by excluding thrombus on transoesophageal echocardiography before cardioversion, the need for prior anticoagulation could be safely avoided. Patients treated in this manner had similar rates of thromboembolism as those treated with the standard antithrombotic regimen but their haemorrhage rates were reduced. Transoesophageal echocardiography guided technique also allowed faster cardioversion of patients and resulted in higher initial success rates, although by eight weeks there was no substantial difference in death rates, maintenance of sinus rhythm, or in functional status between the two groups. Transoesophageal echocardiography guided cardioversion is now regarded by many as the optimum approach to cardioversion and is recognised as a suitable alternative to standard practice by the ACCP. This point is included in the recent American Heart Association (AHA)/American College of Cardiology (ACC)/European Society of Cardiology (ESC) guideline recommendations.

Recent trials comparing a "rate control" strategy with a "rhythm control" strategy for persistent atrial fibrillation showed an excess of thromboembolism in the patients randomised to rhythm control (that is—cardioversion), as such events happened in patients successfully cardioverted, the anticoagulation stopped and on recurrence of atrial fibrillation, thromboembolism occurred. Thus, anticoagulation should be considered long term in patients postcardioversion at high risk of stroke and thromboembolim, or high arrhythmia recurrence risk after cardioversion.

The box showing the benefits of anticoagulant treatment in patients with non-rheumatic atrial fibrillation in preventing stroke is adapted from Straus SE, et al. *JAMA* 2002;288:1388. The table showing the rate versus rhythm in atrial fibrillation: ischaemic strokes is adapted from Verheught FWA et al. *J Am Coll Cardiol* 2003;41:130A. The table showing ischaemic stroke in the AFFIRM study is adapted from the AFFIRM Investigators *New Engl J Med* 2002;347:1825-33. The box showing the recommendations for antithrombotic therapy to prevent ischaemic stroke and systemic embolism in patients with atrial fibrillation undergoing cardioversion is adapted from the ACC/AHA/ESC guidelines *Eur Heart J* 2001;22:1852-93

### Rate versus rhythm in atrial fibrillation: ischaemic strokes

| Study | n | Rate control (%) | Rhythm control | Relative ratio (95% CI) | p |
|---|---|---|---|---|---|
| AFFIRM | 4917 | 5.7 | 7.3 | 1.28 (0.95 to 1.72) | 0.12 |
| RACE | 522 | 5.5 | 7.9 | 1.44 (0.75 to 2.78) | 0.44 |
| STAF | 266 | 1.0 | 3.0 | 3.01 (0.35 to 25.30) | 0.52 |
| PIAF | 252 | 0.8 | 0.8 | 1.02 (0.73 to 2.16) | 0.49 |
| Total | 5957 | 5.0 | 6.5 | 1.28 (0.98 to 1.66) | 0.08 |

### Ischaemic stroke in the AFFIRM study

| | Rhythm control | Rate control |
|---|---|---|
| Ischaemic stroke | 84 (7.3%)* | 79 (5.7%)* |
| INR ≥2.0 | 18 (22%) | 24 (30%) |
| INR <2.0 | 17 (20%) | 28 (35%) |
| Not taking warfarin | 48 (58%) | 26 (33%) |
| Atrial fibrillation at time of event | 25 (36%) | 45 (69%) |

*Event rates derived from Kaplan Meier analysis, p = 0.680

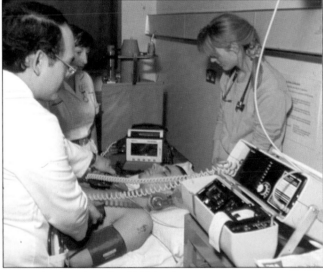

Electrical cardioversion of atrial fibrillation

**Recommendations for antithrombotic therapy to prevent ischaemic stroke and sytemic embolism in patients with atrial fibrillation undergoing cardioversion***

**Class 1**
- Administer anticoagulation therapy regardless of the method (electrical or pharmacological) used to restore sinus rhythm
- Anticoagulate patients with atrial fibrillation lasting more that 48 hours or of unknown duration for at least three to four weeks before and after cardioversion (INR 2.0-3.0)
- Perform immediate cardioversion in patients with acute (recent onset) atrial fibrillation accompanied by symptoms or signs of haemodynamic instability resulting in angina pectoris, myocardial infarction, shock, or pulmonary oedema, without waiting for prior anticoagulation
  - If not contraindicated, administer heparin concurrently by an initial intravenous bolus injection followed by a continuous infusion in a dose adjusted to prolong the activated partial thromboplastin time at 1.5-2.0 times the reference control value
  - Next, provide oral anticoagulation (INR 2.0-3.0) for at least three to four weeks, as for patients who are undergoing elective cardioversion
  - Limited data from recent studies support subcutaneous administration of low molecular weight heparin in this indication
- Screening for the precence of thrombus in the left atrium or left atrial appendage by transoesophageal echocardiography is an alternative to routine preanticoagulation in candidates for cardioversion of atrial fibrillation
  - Anticoagulate patients in whom no thrombus is identified with intravenous unfractionated heparin by an initial bolus injection before cardioversion, followed by a continuous infusion in a dose adjusted to prolong the activated partial thromboplastin time at 1.5-2.0 times the reference control value
  - Next, provide oral anticoagulation (INR 2.0-3.0) for at least three to four weeks, as for patients who are undergoing elective cardioversion
  - Limited data from recent studies support subcutaneous administration of low molecular weight heparin in this indication
  - Treat patients in whom thrombus is identified by transoesophageal echocardiography with oral anticoagulation (INR 2.0-3.0) for at least three to four weeks before and after restoration of sinus rhythm

**Class IIb**
- Cardioversion without transoesophageal echocardiography guidance during the first 48 hours after the onset of atrial fibrillation
  - In these cases, anticoagulation before and after cardioversion is optional, depending on assessment of risk
- Anticoagulate patients with atrial flutter undergoing cardioversion in the same way as for patients with atrial fibrillation

**ACC/AHA Classification**
*Class I*—Conditions for which there is evidence or general agreement or both that a given procedure or treatment if useful and effective
*Class II*—Conditions for which there is conflicting evidence or a divergence of opinion about the usefulness and efficacy of a procedure or treatment
*Class IIa*—Weight of evidence and opinion is in favour of usefulness and efficacy
*ClassIIb*—Usefulness and efficacy is less well established by evidence and opinion
*Class III*—Conditions for which there is evidence or general agreement or both that the procedure or treatment is not useful and in some cases may be harmful

*Data from Fuster V et al. *J Am Cardiol* 2001;38:1231.

**Further reading**
- Rate Control Versus Electrical Cardioversion for Persistent Atrial Fibrillation Study Group. A comparison of rate control and rhythm control in patients with recurrent persistent atrial fibrillation. *New Engl J Med* 2002;347:1834-40
- AFFIRM Investigators. Survival in patients presenting with atrial fibrillation follow up investigation of rhythm management study. *New Engl J Med* 2002;347:1825-33
- Lip GYH. The prothrombotic state in atrial fibrillation: new insights, more questions, and clear answers needed. *Am Heart J* 2000;140:348-50
- Fuster V, Ryden LE, Asinger RW, Cannom DS, Crijns HJ, Frye RL, et al. ACC/AHA/ESC guidelines for the management of patients with atrial fibrillation. A report of the American College of Cardiology, American Heart Association Task Force on practice guidelines and the European society of Cardiology Committee for Practice Guidelines and Policy Conferences developed in collaboration with the North American Society of Pacing and Electrophysiology. *Eur Heart J* 2001;22:1852-923

# 7 Antithrombotic therapy in peripheral vascular disease

Andrew J Makin, Stanley H Silverman, Gregory Y H Lip

Atherosclerotic peripheral vascular disease is symptomatic as intermittent claudication in 2-3% of men and 1-2 % of women aged over 60 years. However, the prevalence of asymptomatic peripheral vascular disease, generally shown by a reduced ankle to brachial systolic pressure index, is three to four times greater. Peripheral vascular disease is also a significant cause of hospital admission, and is an important predicator of cardiovascular mortality. Pain at rest and critical ischaemia are usually the result of progression of atherosclerotic disease, leading to multilevel arterial occlusion. Other causes of arterial insufficiency—including fibromuscular dysplasia, inflammatory conditions, and congenital malformations—are much rarer. Therapeutic objectives in peripheral vascular disease include relieving symptoms and preventing the disease, and any associated events, progressing.

The symptoms of peripheral vascular disease are progressive. A claudicating patient encouraged to exercise tends to report a symptomatic improvement. This effect is generally not accepted to be an improvement in the diseased segment of blood vessel, but the formation of collateral vessels perfusing the ischaemic tissue.

Vasodilating agents, such as naftidrofuryl, have little value in managing claudication and peripheral vascular disease as their effect is small and does not stop progression of the disease. Cilostazol has been shown to increase absolute walking distance in some patients by up to 47%. However, it has no clear antithrombotic effect and has not been shown to stop disease progression.

Unfortunately, not all progression is amenable to improvement and, without the appropriate risk factor management, progression to rest pain and necrosis can be rapid.

## Intermittent claudication

The role of aspirin as an antiplatelet agent has been shown to be beneficial beyond doubt. In peripheral vascular disease it reduces the frequency of thrombotic events in the peripheral arteries and reduces overall cardiovascular mortality in claudicating patients. The dose of aspirin has been the subject of some debate, but 81-325 mg daily has been shown to be of value. Larger doses have no apparent additional benefit but increase the risk of adverse effects. Aspirin has been shown to reduce the progression of atherosclerosis in a few trials, but this remains unsubstantiated.

The role of dipyridamole remains controversial. Several small studies have shown the benefit of giving it in conjunction with aspirin, but it is uncertain if dipyridamole alone is superior to aspirin.

In aspirin intolerant patients there is now a clear role for clopidogrel 75 mg once a day. This is as effective as aspirin in preventing cardiovascular events. If a thrombotic event has occurred (whether the patient is taking aspirin or not) there may be an advantage in using clopidogrel to prevent further events, especially in peripheral vascular disease.

In non-critical peripheral ischaemia, there is no indication for warfarin treatment as the complexities of management and bleeding risks seem to far outweigh the benefits, unless the

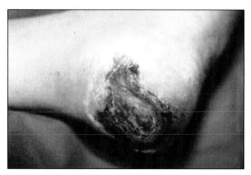
Ischaemic ulcer on foot

**Antithrombotic therapy in peripheral vascular disease**

| Clinical problem | Antithrombotic therapy of choice |
|---|---|
| Intermittent claudication | Aspirin (to reduce risk of stroke and myocardial infarction) Clopidogrel |
| Diabetes | Aspirin (to reduce risk of stroke and myocardial infarction) Clopidogrel |
| Embolic arterial occlusion | Intravenous heparin and emergency surgical intervention |
| Acute on chronic arterial occlusion | Heparin and angioplasty, intra-arterial thrombolysis or early surgery |
| Intraoperative anticoagulation during vascular surgery | Heparin |
| Infrainguinal vein bypass and infrainguinal prosthetic bypass | Aspirin (to reduce risk of stroke and myocardial infarction) Clopidogrel (if unable to take aspirin) |
| Infrainguinal bypass at high thrombotic risk | Aspirin or consider warfarin |
| Carotid endarterectomy | Aspirin or clopidogrel |
| Symptomatic carotid stenosis and too unwell for surgery | Consider warfarin or aspirin plus dipyridamole |

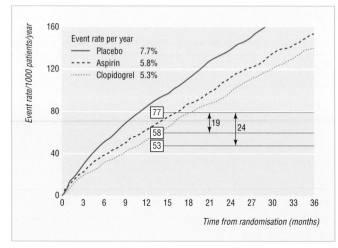
Survival curve from CAPRIE study showing the benefits of aspirin and clopidogrel on vascular events, with placebo rates from the Antiplatelet Trialists' Collaboration

patient has concomitant problems needing anticoagulation such as atrial fibrillation.

# Critical ischaemia

Rest pain and gangrene are markers of critical ischaemia. This is nearly always the result of extensive vessel occlusion with absent pedal pulses. The patient will almost certainly be immobile because of pain and arterial insufficiency making walking impossible. These patients need prophylaxis against venous thromboembolism.

Patients giving a short history of rest pain of sudden onset require full, immediate anticoagulation with low molecular weight heparin or intravenous unfractionated heparin (the latter with a target activated partial prothrombin time (APTT) ratio of 1.5-2.5). Warfarin should be avoided initially until investigations and possible interventions are complete.

Patients with chronic, progressive pain at rest also need full anticoagulation. Although the evidence is limited, these patients are often treated with warfarin to prevent progression, especially if remedial surgery is not possible. The international normalised ratio (INR) should be kept in the range of 2-3.

Acute thromboembolic occlusion of the peripheral arteries requires immediate anticoagulation with intravenous unfractionated heparin to prevent propagation of the thrombus and to guard against further embolism. Surgical intervention or, less commonly, thrombolytic therapy is indicated. Once the embolus has been cleared, the source needs to be investigated and this usually requires treatment with warfarin long term.

# Peripheral artery revascularisation

When the ischaemia reaches a state where peripheral artery revascularisation or reconstruction is necessary, the requirements for antithrombotic therapy change.

Neointimal hyperplasia is a considerable problem in the long term survival of a graft as its consequences (reduced blood flow caused by reduced lumen) in some respects mimic those of the original disease. Hyperplasia of smooth muscle cells can occur along the entire length of a vein graft, but particularly does so at the anastomoses of prosthetic grafts.

Aspirin has no apparent effect on graft survival in humans. One trial showed that low molecular weight heparin had a profound beneficial effect on graft patency, when compared with aspirin and dipyridamole over three months, suggesting that early treatment with low molecular weight heparin suppresses neointimal hyperplasia. In the United Kingdom most low molecular weight heparins have licences only for 14 days'

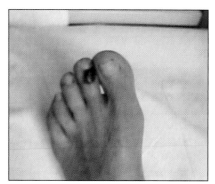
Gangrenous toe indicating critical ischaemia

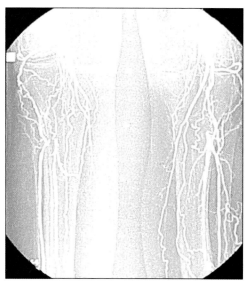
Peripheral angiogram showing chronic occlusions with multiple collateral vessels

## Risk of thrombosis with different vein grafts

| Site of proximal anastomosis | Site of distal anastomosis | Graft material | Other factors | Thrombotic risk | Recommended antithrombotic therapy |
|---|---|---|---|---|---|
| Aorta | Iliac or femoral | Prosthetic | | Low | Antiplatelet* |
| Axilla | Femoral | Prosthetic | | Medium | Antiplatelet |
| Femoral | Popliteal (above knee joint) | Vein | | Low | Antiplatelet* |
| | | Prosthetic | | Low | Antiplatelet* |
| | Distal (below knee) | Vein | Good flow (>100 ml/min) and good distal arteries | Medium | Antiplatelet |
| | | | Poor flow (<50 ml/min) or poor distal arteries | High | Antiplatelet Consider warfarin |
| | | Prosthetic | | High | Antiplatelet Consider warfarin |

*Antiplatelet therapy not indicated for graft survival but recommended as prophylaxis against cardiovascular events

treatment, and, until more data are available, the prolonged use of low molecular weight heparin cannot be recommended.

### Infrainguinal bypass

Antiplatelet treatment has no beneficial role for graft patency in short (femoral-popliteal) bypass with native vein grafts because these are high flow and non-thrombogenic. None the less, aspirin has been shown to reduce all cardiovascular end points in patients with peripheral vascular disease, and so should be continued. Anticoagulation with warfarin has not been shown to be of benefit.

Patients with prosthetic femoral-popliteal bypass are a different consideration. Taking aspirin with dipyridamole reduces platelet accumulation at the anastomosis. Starting antiplatelet treatment preoperatively leads to improved patency rates, especially in "high risk" (low flow, prosthetic) grafts once the increased complication rate of postoperative wound haematoma has passed. Again, aspirin (with or without dipyridamole) is recommended.

High risk grafts need to be dealt with cautiously. All patients should continue taking aspirin (or clopidogrel). The use of warfarin needs to be judged carefully. In cases of poor run off, marginal quality vein, and previous graft failure, oral anticoagulation has been shown to improve primary patency and limb salvage rates with a target INR of 2-3. If this is being considered then full heparinisation should begin immediately after the operation while oral anticoagulation is started. Naturally, older patients are more likely to have bleeding complications, including intracranial haemorrhage, and this should be considered.

### Aortoiliac and aortofemoral grafts

Large aortoiliac and aortofemoral grafts are at low risk of thrombosis. Primary patency rates of 80-90% can be expected at five to ten years. Thus, specific antithrombotic therapy is not indicated. However, once again, the presence of peripheral vascular disease needs antiplatelet therapy to reduce all cardiovascular end points.

### Percutaneous transluminal angioplasty

Almost all patients undergoing percutaneous transluminal angioplasty have atherosclerotic peripheral vascular disease. As such, they should all be treated with aspirin or clopidogrel.

Studies with radiolabelled platelets have found substantial platelet accumulation at the sites of angioplasty, and antiplatelet treatment reduces this. In coronary angiography, this treatment has been shown to reduce the incidence of new thrombus at the site of the angioplasty. However, in similar coronary artery studies, antiplatelet treatment has no effect on restenosis compared with placebo. It is unclear how these results will extrapolate to peripheral angioplasty, and there are insufficient data to make recommendations in peripheral vascular disease.

Similarly there have not been enough studies to recommend the use of dipyridamole, ticlopidine, or clopidogrel as an adjunct to aspirin. Although the long term use of antiplatelet drugs is not known to have any long term effect on restenosis, the drug should be used to prevent cardiovascular mortality in patients undergoing percutaneous transluminal angioplasty.

### Carotid stenosis

Evidence for treatment of asymptomatic carotid stenosis of greater than 50% is unclear. One trial showed no reduction in stroke rate in patients treated with aspirin for two to three years. However, it is increasingly accepted that atherosclerosis affects all arteries to a greater or lesser extent. With this in mind, and

---

**Problems in patients undergoing infrainguinal bypass**

- The thrombogenic characteristics of prosthetic graft materials
- The poor flow states associated with some grafts, for example, long bypasses passing over the knee joint
- The medium to long term complication of neointimal hyperplasia

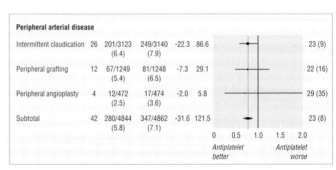

Meta-analysis from the Antithrombotic Trialists' Collaboration showing the benefits of antiplatelet treatment in patients with peripheral vascular disease

**Among high risk patients, antiplatelet treatment reduces the combined outcome of any serious vascular event by about a quarter, non-fatal myocardial infarction by a third, non-fatal stroke by a quarter, and vascular mortality by a sixth (with no apparent adverse effect on other deaths)**

---

**Suggestions from the Antithrombotic Trialists' Collaboration**

- Clopidogrel reduced serious vascular events by 10% compared with aspirin, which was similar to the 12% reduction observed with its analogue ticlopidine
- Addition of dipyridamole to aspirin produced no significant further reduction in vascular events compared with aspirin alone

the evidence for using aspirin in lower limb atherosclerosis, it is still recommended that these patients have antiplatelet treatment to prevent all cardiovascular events.

Treating patients who have had a transient ischaemic attack or known ischaemic stroke with aspirin has clear benefit as shown by the Antiplatelet Trialists' Collaboration. The dose is not clear, but 81-325 mg should be effective without unacceptable bleeding risk. Clopidogrel (75 mg daily) is recommended for aspirin intolerant patients. Limited evidence shows that the combination of aspirin and dipyridamole (400 mg daily) may be more beneficial to these patients than aspirin alone.

Inadequate data exist on the use of warfarin in symptomatic carotid stenosis, and so this cannot be recommended because of possible bleeding complications.

Carotid endarterectomy is the treatment of choice for all symptomatic carotid stenosis. Aspirin treatment should be continued in the perioperative period to prevent platelet deposition at the site of the endarterectomy and thus reduce intraoperative and postoperative stroke. Platelet deposition is known to start immediately after the operation, and aspirin started in the first few postoperative days seems to provide much less benefit. In patients with symptomatic disease who are not undergoing endarterectomy antiplatelet therapy is essential to reduce the incidence of ischaemic stroke. Again, warfarin should not be used as not enough evidence exists. In all patients with cerebrovascular or carotid disease, antiplatelet therapy is recommended at all stages to decrease the risk of cardiovascular events.

## Further reading

- Jackson MR, Clagett GP. Antithrombotic therapy in peripheral arterial occlusive disease. *Chest* 2001;119:293-9S
- CAPRIE Steering Committee. A randomised, blinded, trial of clopidogrel versus aspirin in patients at risk of ischaemic events (CAPRIE). *Lancet* 1996;348:1329-39
- Antiplatelet Trialists' Collaboration. Collaborative overview of randomised trials of antiplatelet therapy I: prevention of death, myocardial infarction, and stroke by prolonged antiplatelet therapy in various categories of patients. *BMJ* 1994;308:81-106
- Antiplatelet Trialists' Collaboration. Collaborative overview of randomised trials of antiplatelet therapy II: maintenance of vascular graft or arterial patency by antiplatelet therapy. *BMJ* 1994;308:159-68
- Antithrombotic Trialists' Collaboration. Collaborative meta-analysis of randomised trials of antiplatelet therapy for prevention of death, myocardial infarction and stroke in high risk patients. *BMJ* 2002;324:71-86

The survival curve from the CAPRIE study is adapted from CAPRIE Steering Committee, *Lancet* 1996;348:1329-39. The table showing the graft risk of thrombosis and the table of antithrombotic therapy in peripheral vascular disease are adapted from Jackson MR, Clagett GP, *Chest* 2001;119: 293-9S. The meta-analysis showing the benefits of antiplatelet treatment in patients with peripheral vascular disease is adapted from the Antithrombotic Trialist's Collaboration, *BMJ* 2002;324:71-86.

# 8   Antithrombotic therapy for cerebrovascular disorders

Gregory Y H Lip, Sridhar Kamath, Robert G Hart

Stroke remains one of the leading causes of death and disability throughout the world. It is the third commonest cause of death in developed countries, exceeded only by coronary artery disease and cancer.

The incidence of stroke is 1-2 cases in 1000 people a year in the Western world, and is probably slightly higher among African-Caribbeans than other ethnic groups. Cerebrovascular disorders are uncommon in people aged <40 years, but there is a definite increase with age, with an incidence of 10 cases in 1000 people aged >75 in a year. Stroke is slightly more common in men, but women tend to have a poorer prognosis because of a higher mean age at onset. The incidence of stroke has been declining in recent decades in many Western countries because of better population control of hypertension, smoking, and other risk factors. However, the absolute number of strokes continues to increase because of the ageing population, which is predicted to peak in 2015. Thus, the present annual incidence of 700 000 strokes in the United States is expected to rise to 1 100 000 in 2015, without further advances in prevention.

About 80-85% of the strokes are ischaemic, with the rest primarily haemorrhagic. Even among patients with ischaemic stroke, there is much heterogeneity in aetiological and pathophysiological factors contributing to the disease.

Atherosclerosis of the major cerebral vessels probably accounts for most ischaemic strokes, either as thrombotic occlusion at the site of atherosclerotic plaques or atherogenic embolism. Embolism from a source in the heart (cardioembolic stroke) and lipohyalinosis of the penetrating small cerebral vessels (lacunar stroke) account for a substantial proportion of ischaemic strokes. In many patients the aetiology remains unknown. The major risk factors for ischaemic stroke include old age, male sex, obesity, hypertension, diabetes, and tobacco smoking.

## Management of acute ischaemic stroke

The principles of management of patients with ischaemic stroke include slowing the progression of stroke, decreasing the recurrence of stroke, decreasing death and disability, preventing deep vein thrombosis and pulmonary embolism, and suppressing fever, managing hypertension and controlling glucose levels.

### Antiplatelet treatment

Aspirin is the only antiplatelet drug evaluated for the treatment of acute ischaemic stroke and is recommended early in the management at a dose of 160-325 mg daily. Two major randomised trials (the international stroke trial (IST) and the Chinese acute stroke trial (CAST)) have shown that starting daily aspirin promptly (<48 hours after the start rather than the end of the hospital stay) in patients with suspected acute ischaemic stroke reduces the immediate risk of further stroke or death in hospital, and the overall risk of death and dependency at six months later. About 10 deaths or recurrent strokes are avoided in every 1000 patients treated with aspirin in the first few weeks after an ischaemic stroke.

The benefit of aspirin is seen in a wide range of patients irrespective of age, sex, atrial fibrillation, blood pressure, stroke subtype, and computed tomographic findings. In IST 300 mg of

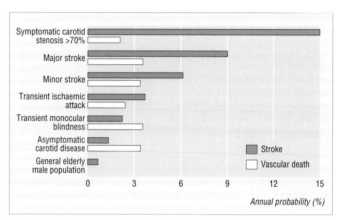

Annual risk of stroke or vascular death among patients in various high risk subgroups

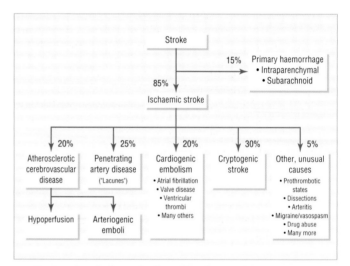

Classification of stroke by mechanism, with estimates of the frequency of various categories of abnormalities

---

**Pathophysiological classification of stroke**

**Thrombosis**
- Atherosclerosis
- Vasculitis
- Thrombophilic disorders
- Drug abuse such as cocaine, amphetamines

**Embolism**
- From the heart
- From the major cerebrovascular vessels
- Unknown source

**Lipohyalinolysis**
- Small penetrating arteries

**Vasospasm**
- Migraine
- Subarachnoid haemorrhage

**Dissection**
- Spontaneous
- Traumatic

---

aspirin was used and in CAST 160 mg. Thus, the two studies show that giving aspirin early in acute stroke is safe, although side effects should always be considered. Other trials have shown that continuing treatment with low dose aspirin gives protection in the longer term. Until further evidence is available, however, aspirin should be withheld from patients receiving other forms of anticoagulant (except low dose heparin (5000 IU twice daily)) or thrombolytic treatment (and for 24 hours after finishing treatment).

The results of the IST and CAST studies apply chiefly to patients who had a computed tomography scan to exclude intracranial haemorrhage. A meta-analysis of subgroups from the trials showed that aspirin was safe and beneficial. Even among patients who did not have a computed tomogram and patients with haemorrhagic stroke, aspirin treatment did not result in net hazard. Thus, aspirin can be started in patients with suspected ischaemic stroke even when computed tomography is not available immediately.

## Anticoagulation treatment

Heparin is not routinely recommended for patients with acute ischaemic stroke. There are no randomised trials supporting the use of standard doses of heparin (for example > 10 000 IU daily) even in patients with acute stroke and risk factors for recurrent events. The risk:benefit ratio of heparin administration is narrow, ill defined, and probably depends on the pathophysiological subtype of stroke and the factors that predispose to haemorrhage. For patients with atrial fibrillation and acute ischaemic stroke, there seems to be no net benefit from standard dose heparin (aspirin should be given immediately, then warfarin (INR 2.0-3.0) started for secondary prevention as soon as the patient is medically stable). However, a subgroup analysis from IST showed that in acute ischaemic stroke low dose heparin (5000 IU twice daily) reduced death and recurrence, especially if combined with aspirin, and it is indicated if appreciable leg weakness is present for prevention of venous thromboembolism.

No particular benefit was observed in ischaemic stroke in the vertebrobasilar region with anticoagulation at six months. Trials with low molecular weight heparins or heparinoids have yielded contradictory (but generally negative) results, and they are not recommended for use at the moment.

## Thrombolytic treatment

Thrombolytic treatment for acute ischaemic stroke has been in vogue since its immense benefit was seen with myocardial infarction. The National Institute of Neurological Disorders and Stroke (NINDS) rtPA Study Group trial showed that recombinant tissue plasminogen activator administered within three hours of onset of acute cerebral infarct at a dose of 0.9 mg/kg (maximum 90 mg) given over an hour under strict treatment protocols increased the likelihood of minimal or no disability at three months by at least 30%. This benefit was seen in all stroke patients. Recombinant tissue plasminogen activator is licensed for treating acute cerebral infarct in several countries. However, the risk:benefit ratio is narrow because of substantial risk of intracerebral haemorrhage, and the need to start treatment (after computed tomographic assessment) within three hours of stroke onset severely restricts the number of patients who can be treated.

Streptokinase is not approved for use in acute cerebral infarct because of the results of three large trials, which were terminated early due to excessive bleeding. These trials used streptokinase at a dose of 1.5 million units given more than three hours after stroke onset. Intra-arterial thrombolytic treatment for patients with large artery occlusions (such as of

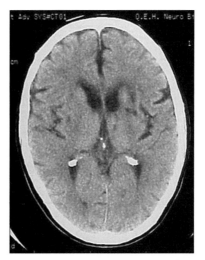

Computed tomogram of the brain showing lacunar infarcts in the anterior limb of the left internal capsule

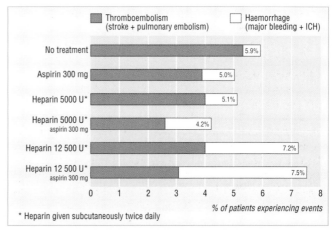

Thromboembolic and major haemorrhagic events in the International Stroke Trial. ICH=intracranial haemorrhage

---

### Cardiac disorders predisposing to stroke

**Major risk**
- Atrial fibrillation
- Prosthetic mechanical heart valve
- Mitral stenosis
- Severe left ventricular dysfunction with mobile left ventricular thrombus
- Recent myocardial infarction
- Infective endocarditis

**Minor risk***
- Mitral annular calcification
- Mitral valve prolapse
- Patent foramen ovale
- Calcific aortic stenosis
- Atrial septal aneurysm

*Occasionally can cause cardioembolic stroke, but the risk of initial stroke is low and often unrelated when identified during the evaluation of patients with cerebral ischaemia

the internal carotid artery, middle cerebral artery, or basilarartery) remains investigational. In the United Kingdom, thrombolytic treatment is not licensed for treatment of stroke, pending results from ongoing clinical trials (for example, IST-3).

# Stroke prevention

In broad terms, antiplatelet agents are more effective in cerebrovascular atherogenic strokes, and anticoagulants are more effective in primary and secondary prophylaxis against cardioembolic stroke.

## Antiplatelet agents

Among patients with vascular disorders (such as coronary artery disease, previous stroke or transient ischaemic attack, and peripheral vascular disease) antiplatelet agents substantially reduce the incidence of non-fatal stroke, non-fatal myocardial infarction, vascular mortality, and composite end point of stroke, myocardial infarction, and vascular death.

A variety of antiplatelet drugs with varying mechanisms of action are used to minimise stroke in patients at high risk. These include aspirin (irreversible inhibitor of cyclo-oxygenase), clopidogrel (which inhibits adenosine diphosphate induced platelet aggregation) and dipyridamole (precise mechanism of action not yet clear). Aspirin remains the most commonly used antiplatelet drug, partly because of its cost effectiveness.

Aspirin is effective for stroke prevention in doses ranging from 30 mg/day to 1300 mg/day. Its beneficial effect is seen in all age groups and sexes. The European stroke prevention study II (ESPS II) showed that a combination of aspirin and dipyridamole (sustained release 200 mg tablets twice daily) significantly reduced the risk of stroke and all vascular events compared with aspirin alone. An important ongoing trial (ESPRIT) is seeking to replicate these results.

Clopidogrel is a newer thienopyridine derivative without the adverse effect profile of ticlopidine. The CAPRIE (clopidogrel versus asprin in patients at risk of ischaemic events) study showed that clopidogrel is slightly more effective than aspirin in reducing the combined outcome of stroke, myocardial infarction, and vascular death among patients with atherosclerotic vascular disease. Although clopidogrel seems to be as safe as aspirin, it is considerably more expensive, and it remains to be seen whether its use in routine practice is cost effective. Its use is justified in patients who are intolerant to aspirin or who develop a stroke while taking aspirin.

## Anticoagulation treatment

Anticoagulation in the form of warfarin has a role in a variety of cardiac disorders in primary and secondary prevention of stroke. Cardiac disorders that predispose to stroke and unequivocally seem to benefit from anticoagulation therapy include atrial fibrillation (with additional risk factors putting patients at moderate to high risk), mitral stenosis (with or without atrial fibrillation), and mechanical valve prosthesis. In contrast, recent randomised trials (SPIRIT, WARSS) did not show advantages of warfarin over aspirin for secondary prevention of non-cardioembolic brain ischaemia. At present, warfarin should not be used routinely for patients with common causes of non-cardioembolic stroke, pending results from ongoing randomised trials.

**Risk factors for haemorrhagic transformation of ischaemic stroke**
- Hypertension
- Concomitant use of two or more antiplatelet or antithrombotic therapies
- Major early infarct signs on pretreatment computed tomography, including brain oedema and mass effect
- Severe neurological deficit

**Details of the second European stroke prevention study (ESPS-II)**
- Randomised, placebo controlled, double blind trial of aspirin (50 mg), dipyridamole (400 mg), or both versus placebo
- Two year follow up of >6600 patients (secondary prevention of stroke)

| Placebo compared with: | Aspirin alone | Dipyridamole alone | Aspirin + dipyridamole |
|---|---|---|---|
| Reduction of stroke risk | 18% (P=0.013) | 16% (P=0.015) | 37% (P<0.001) |
| Reduction of risk of stroke or death | 13% (P=0.016) | 15% (P=0.015) | 24% (P<0.001) |

- Clear additive benefit in stroke reduction (36%) when aspirin and dipyridamole were used in combination

## Further reading

- Adams HP. Emergency use of anticoagulation for treatment of patients with ischemic stroke. *Stroke* 2002;33:856-61
- Antithrombotic Trialists' Collaboration. Collaborative meta-analysis of randomised trials of antiplatelet therapy for prevention of death, myocardial infarction, and stroke in high-risk patients. *BMJ* 2002;324:71-86
- Albers GW, Amarenco P, Easton JD, Sacco RL, Teal P. Antithrombotic and thrombolytic therapy for ischemic stroke. *Chest* 2001;119:300–20S
- Atkinson RP, DeLemos C. Acute ischemic stroke management. *Thromb Res* 2000;98:V97-111
- CAPRIE Steering Committee. A randomised, blinded trial of clopidogrel versus aspirin in patients at risk of ischaemic events (CAPRIE). *Lancet* 1996;348:1329-39
- CAST Collaborative Group. CAST: randomised placebo-controlled trial of early aspirin use in 20 000 patients with acute ischaemic stroke. *Lancet* 1997;349:1641-9
- International Stroke Trials Collaborative Group. IST: a randomised trial of aspirin, subcutaneous heparin, both, or neither among 19 435 patients with acute ischaemic stroke. *Lancet* 1997;349:1569-81
- Mohr JP, Thompson JLP, Lazar RM, Levin B, Sacco RL, Furie KL, et al for the Warfarin-Aspirin Recurrent Stroke Study Group. A comparison of warfarin and aspirin for the prevention of recurrent ischemic stroke. *N Engl J Med* 2002;345:1444-51

The flow diagram showing a classification of stroke by mechanism with estimates of the frequency of various categories of abnormalities is adapted from Albers GW et al, *Chest* 2001;119:300-20. Annual risk of stroke or vascular death among patients in various high risk subgroups is adapted from Wilterdink and Easton, *Arch Neurol* 1992;49:857-63. The figure showing thromboembolic and major haemorrhagic events in the IST is adapted from IST Collaborative Group. *Lancet* 1997;349:1569-81.

# 9 Valvar heart disease and prosthetic heart valves

Ira Goldsmith, Alexander G G Turpie, Gregory Y H Lip

Thromboembolism and anticoagulant related bleeding are major life threatening complications in patients with valvar heart disease and those with prosthetic heart valves. In these patients effective and safe antithrombotic therapy is indicated to reduce the risks of thromboembolism while keeping bleeding complications to a minimum.

## Assessment

Risk factors that increase the incidence of systemic embolism must be considered when defining the need for starting antithrombotic therapy in patients with cardiac valvar disease and prosthetic heart valves. These factors include age, smoking, hypertension, diabetes, hyperlipidaemia, type and severity of valve lesion, presence of atrial fibrillation, heart failure or low cardiac output, size of the left atrium (over 50 mm on echocardiography), previous thromboembolism, and abnormalities of the coagulation system including hepatic failure.

Secondly, the type, number, and location of prostheses implanted must be considered. For example, mechanical prostheses are more thrombogenic than bioprostheses or homografts, and hence patients with mechanical valves require lifelong anticoagulant therapy. However, the intensity of treatment varies according to the type of mechanical prosthesis implanted. First generation mechanical valves, namely the Starr-Edwards caged ball valve and Bjork-Shiley standard valves, have a high thromboembolic risk; single tilting disc valves have an intermediate thromboembolic risk; and the newer (second and third generation) bileaflet valves have low thromboembolic risks.

In patients with a bioprosthesis in sinus rhythm, antithrombotic therapy with an antiplatelet drug may suffice, whereas patients with homografts in sinus rhythm may not need any antithrombotic therapy. Thromboembolic events are commoner with prosthetic mitral valves than aortic valves and in patients with double replacement valves compared with those with single replaced valves. Moreover, the risk of thromboembolic events is greatest in the first three months after implantation.

## Choice of antithrombotic agent

Warfarin is the most used oral anticoagulant, and its dose is guided by achieving a target international normalised ratio (INR) range. The use of heparin is confined to short periods when anticoagulant cover is needed and oral anticoagulants are stopped. The dose of heparin is adjusted to achieve at least twice normal level of activated partial thromboplastin time (APTT) regardless of cardiac rhythm and type or position of prosthesis. Fixed weight-adjusted low molecular weight heparin may be used as an alternative to unfractionated heparin. Antiplatelet drugs, such as low dose aspirin or dipyridamole, are used in patients with bioprosthesis in sinus rhythm and in addition to anticoagulants in the high risk patients with mechanical valves.

Patients with mechanical valves and those with bioprostheses and associated risk factors require lifelong anticoagulant cover. In patients with a bioprosthetic valve in sinus rhythm anticoagulant cover with warfarin for the first three postoperative months may suffice, followed by low dose aspirin treatment for life. Alternatively, some surgeons give only low dose aspirin after

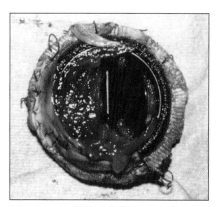

Valve thrombosis of a bileaflet prosthetic mitral valve

---

**Considerations for antithrombotic therapy in patients with valve disease**

- Assessment of risk for thromboembolic events, which may be patient related or valve prosthesis related
- Indications for starting treatment
- Choice of antithrombotic agent
- Duration of treatment and optimal therapeutic range
- Antithrombotic therapy in special circumstances (surgical procedures, pregnancy, and resistance to oral anticoagulants)
- Management of treatment failures and complications

---

**Types of prosthetic valves and thrombogenicity**

| Type of valve | Model | Thrombogenicity |
|---|:---:|:---:|
| *Mechanical* | | |
| Caged ball | Starr-Edwards | + + + + |
| Single tilting disc | Bjork-Shiley, Medtronic Hall | + + + |
| Bileaflet | St Jude Medical, Sorin Bicarbon, Carbomedics | + + |
| *Bioprosthetic* | | |
| Heterografts | Carpentier-Edwards, Tissue Med (Aspire), Hancock II | + to + + |
| Homografts | | + |

---

**Risk factors for patients with bioprostheses include previous thromboembolic events, atrial fibrillation, enlarged left atrial cavity, and severe cardiac failure**

surgery in patients with bioprostheses in sinus rhythm (providing aspirin is not contraindicated). Patients with homografts usually do not require any antithrombotic therapy.

# Indications for antithrombotic therapy

### Native valve disease
Oral anticoagulant treatment is indicated in all patients who have established or paroxysmal atrial fibrillation with native valve disease regardless of the nature or severity of the valve disease. In patients with mitral stenosis in sinus rhythm, treatment is guided by the severity of stenosis, the patient's age, size of the left atrium, and the presence of spontaneous echocontrast or echocardiographic evidence of left atrial appendage thrombus. In these patients a target INR of 2.5 (range 2-3) is recommended. Similarly, in patients with mitral regurgitation treatment is indicated in the presence of congestive cardiac failure, marked cardiomegaly with low cardiac output, and an enlarged left atrium. In the absence of cardiac failure, previous thromboemboli, or heart failure, antithrombotic therapy is not indicated in patients with isolated aortic or tricuspid valve disease.

Mitral valve prolapse per se does not require anticoagulant cover, although sometimes aspirin is recommended because of the association with cerebrovascular events.

### Percutaneous balloon valvuloplasty
In patients with mitral stenosis, the presence or absence of left atrial thrombus is first confirmed by transoesophageal echocardiography. In the presence of thrombus, valvuloplasty is deferred and anticoagulant treatment started for two months before the procedure, with a target INR range of 2-3. In the absence of atrial thrombus but in the presence of risk factors—namely, previous thromboembolism, enlarged left atrium, spontaneous echocontrast, or atrial fibrillation—oral anticoagulant treatment should be started a month before the procedure.

During the procedure, intravenous heparin (2000-5000 IU bolus) should be given to all patients immediately after trans-septal catheterisation. After the procedure, subcutaneous heparin should be given for 24 hours and oral anticoagulant treatment restarted 24 hours after the procedure in patients with risk factors, especially in the presence of atrial fibrillation or spontaneous echocontrast.

Patients in sinus rhythm who are undergoing aortic valvuloplasty do not need long term anticoagulant treatment. However, treatment with heparin during the procedure is required.

### Mitral valve repair
After mitral valve repair, oral anticoagulation (target INR 2.5) is needed for the first six weeks to three months, and thereafter treatment is guided by the presence or absence of risk factors such as atrial fibrillation, heart failure, and enlarged left atrium.

### Heart valve replacement
Antithrombotic therapy in patients with replaced heart valves is guided by the type of prosthesis implanted (mechanical or biological), position of the implant, associated risk factors (such as atrial fibrillation), previous thromboembolism, bleeding risk, and the patient's age.

Patients with porcine or pericardial bioprostheses in sinus rhythm may be started on lifelong antiplatelet treatment with low dose aspirin as soon as they can swallow the drugs.

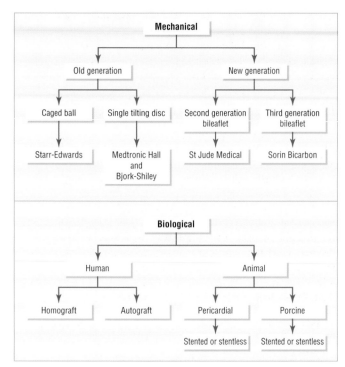

Types of heart valve prostheses

### Comparison of mechanical and biological valve prostheses

| Mechanical | Biological |
|---|---|
| Durable—valves lasting 20-30 years | Limited life span—10% of homografts and 30% of heterografts fail within 10-15 years |
| Thrombogenic—patients require lifelong anticoagulant therapy | Low thrombogenic potential—lifelong anticoagulation is not required |
| Preferred in younger patients with >10-15 years life expectancy | Preferred in older patients with <10-15 years life expectancy |
| Preferred in patients who require lifelong anticoagulant therapy | Preferred in those who cannot (or will not) take lifelong anticoagulant therapy |

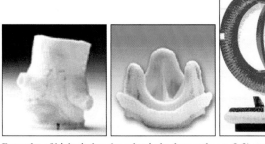

Examples of biological and mechanical valve protheses: (left) stentless porcine valve, (middle) stented porcine valve, (right) Sorin Bicarbon valve

However, many centres start oral anticoagulant treatment the day after implantation, maintaining an INR range of 2-3 for the first three months. Lifelong anticoagulant treatment is recommended for patients with associated risk factors. These factors are previous thromboembolism, left atrial thrombus, marked cardiomegaly, heart failure, dilated left atrium, or spontaneous echocontrast.

Patients with mechanical heart valves require lifelong anticoagulant treatment, and patients with first generation valves (with the highest thromboembolic risk) need a higher target INR than patients with single tilting disc prostheses (intermediate thromboembolic risk) or the newer bileaflet prosthesis (lower thromboembolic risk).

Most centres start (or restart) oral anticoagulant treatment the day after implantation, with or without heparinisation. As the thromboembolic risk is highest in the early postoperative period, it is advisable to give heparin and to continue it until the oral anticoagulant treatment achieves the target INR. The dose of heparin should be adjusted to achieve twice the normal level of APTT regardless of cardiac rhythm and type or position of the valve.

The European and North American guidelines have minor differences. The duration of antithrombotic therapy also varies according to a number of factors. Lifelong anticoagulant treatment is indicated for patients with mechanical valves and those with bioprosthetic valves or native valve disease with additional risk factors.

# Antithrombotic therapy in special circumstances

Modification of anticoagulant treatment may be required in patients who have prosthetic valves and are undergoing non-cardiac surgical procedures, who are are pregnant, or who have resistance to oral anticoagulants.

### Surgical procedures

For minor procedures, such as certain dental surgery or cryotherapy, where blood loss is expected to be minimal and easily manageable, anticoagulant treatment may be continued. After dental extraction bleeding can be stopped with oral tranexamic acid (4.8%) mouth wash. However, before a planned minor surgical procedure, the INR should be adjusted to between 1.5 and 2.0. This can be achieved by stopping or adjusting oral anticoagulant treatment one to three days before the procedure depending on the drug used. In most cases, resumption of oral anticoagulant treatment is possible on the same day as the procedure, and interim heparin treatment is not needed. Patients undergoing endoscopic procedures and in whom an endoscopic biopsy is anticipated should be managed in the same way as patients needing major non-cardiac surgical procedures.

For major non-cardiac surgical procedures, in which there is a substantial risk of bleeding, anticoagulation should be discontinued for several days (generally four to five days) before surgery and the INR should be normalised at 1.0. The risk of thromboembolism increases, and so interim heparin treatment should be given in a dose that prolongs the APTT to twice the control value. However, heparin should be stopped in time to bring the APTT down to near normal at the time of operation and resumed as soon as possible postoperatively. An alternative approach would be to use therapeutic fixed weight-adjusted doses of low molecular weight heparin.

## Intensity of anticoagulation guidelines for Europe

| | European Society of Cardiology 1995 INR range | British Society of Haematology 1998 INR target |
|---|---|---|
| *Mechanical valves** | | |
| Aortic: | | |
| First generation | 3.0-4.5 | 3.5 |
| Second generation | 2.5-3.0 | 3.5† |
| Third generation | 2.5-3.0 | 3.5† |
| Mitral | 3.0-3.5 | 3.5 |
| *Bioprosthetic valves* | | |
| In sinus rhythm: | | |
| Aortic | 2.5-3.0 for three months | No anticoagulation‡ |
| Mitral | 3.0-3.5 for three months. No anticoagulation after three months | 2.5 for three months. No anticoagulation after three months |
| In atrial fibrillation: | | |
| Rheumatic valvar heart disease | 3.0-4.5 | 2.5 |
| Patients with recurrent emboli under adequate anticoagulation | 3.0-4.5 + 100 mg aspirin | — |
| Non-valvar atrial fibrillation with risk factors | 2.0-3.0 | 2.5 |

*First generation valves include Starr-Edwards and Bjork-Shiley; second generation valves include St Jude Medical and Medtronic Hall; and third generation valves include the Sorin Bicarbon bileaflet valve
†For second and third generation mechanical aortic valves a target INR of 2.5 is used
‡Low dose aspirin is used by most centres in the United Kingdom

## Intensity of anticoagulation guidelines for North America

| | AHA and ACC 1998 INR range | ACCP 2001 INR (target range) |
|---|---|---|
| *Mechanical valves* | | |
| First, second, and third generation valves: | | |
| Aortic | 2.0-3.0 | 2.5 (2.0-3.0) |
| Mitral | 2.5-3.5 | 3.0 (2.5-3.5) |
| *Bioprosthetic valves* | | |
| In sinus rhythm: | | |
| Aortic | Aspirin 80-100 mg/day | 2.5 (2.0-3.0) for three months |
| Mitral | Aspirin 80-100 mg/day. No anticoagulation after three months | 2.5 (2.0-3.0) for three months |
| In atrial fibrillation: | | |
| Aortic | 2.0-3.0 | 2.5 (2.0-3.0) |
| Mitral | 2.5-3.5 | 2.5 (2.0-3.0) |

AHA = American Heart Association; ACC = American College of Cardiology; ACCP = American College of Chest Physicians

**Pregnancy**

In pregnant women with prosthetic valves, the incidence of thromboembolic complications is increased. Hence, adequate antithrombotic therapy is particularly important. Warfarin use in the first trimester of pregnancy is associated with a substantial risk of embryopathy and fetal death, and so warfarin should be stopped when a patient is trying to become pregnant or when pregnancy is detected. Instead, twice daily subcutaneous unfractionated heparin should be given to prolong the APTT to twice the control value, and this treatment may be continued until delivery. Alternatively, unfractionated heparin may be given until the thirteenth week of pregnancy, then a switch made to warfarin treatment until the middle of the third trimester. Then warfarin can be stopped and unfractionated heparin resumed until delivery. Because low dose aspirin is safe for mother and child, it may be used in conjunction with anticoagulant treatment in women at high risk of thromboembolism. However, low molecular weight heparin (which does not cross the placental barrier) may be an alternative to unfractionated heparin in this setting, although there are limited data on its efficacy or safety in pregnancy. Other pregnancy related issues are discussed in chapter 14.

---

**Management of temporary interruption of oral anticoagulants**

- Discontinue oral anticoagulation five days before the procedure
- Measure INR three days before procedure
  If INR $<2$ start low molecular weight heparin in therapeutic doses
  If INR $>2.5$ consider giving Vitamin $K_1$ 1-2 mg orally and start low molecular weight heparin in therapeutic doses. Repeat INR measurement the day before procedure
- Continue low molecular weight heparin until evening before procedure (last injection not less than 12 hours preprocedure)
- Restart warfarin night of or day after procedure
- Restart low molecular weight heparin 12-24 hours after procedure and when haemostasis is established

---

**Indications for lifelong oral anticoagulation in valve disease**

- Mechanical prostheses
- Chronic or paroxysmal atrial fibrillation in the presence of native valve disease, bioprosthesis, valve repair, or valvuloplasty
- Native valve disease and previous thromboembolism
- Mitral valve stenosis, irrespective of rhythm, in association with high transmitral valve gradient, left atrial thrombus, spontaneous echocontrast, large left atrium ($>50$ mm), low cardiac output, or congestive heart failure

---

**Further reading**

- Bonow RO, Carobello D, de Leon AC, Edmunds LH Jr, Fedderly BJ, Freed MD, et al. ACC/AHA guidelines for the management of patients with valvular heart disease. *J Am Coll Cardiol* 1998; 32:1486-8
- Gohlke-Barwölf C. Anticoagulation in valvular heart disease: new aspects and management during non-cardiac surgery. *Heart* 2000;84:567-72
- Haemostasis and Thrombosis Task Force of the British Society for Haematology. Guidelines for prevention of thromboembolic events in valvular heart disease. *Eur Heart J* 1995;16:1320-30

# 10 Antithrombotic therapy in myocardial infarction and stable angina

Gregory Y H Lip, Bernard S P Chin, Neeraj Prasad

## Acute Q wave myocardial infarction

The use of thrombolytic treatment in acute myocardial infarction is now established beyond doubt. However, primary angioplasty is now proved to be an effective alternative and is used increasingly in preference to thrombolysis in many centres worldwide.

### Thrombolytic treatment

Current key issues relate to the clinical situations in which thrombolysis may be beneficial or contraindicated. For example, all patients with a history suggesting cardiac ischaemia and accompanying electrocardiographic changes indicating acute myocardial infarction should be considered for thrombolysis. However, patients with only ST segment depression on an electrocardiogram or with a normal electrocardiogram do not benefit from thrombolysis, and treatment should therefore be withheld. Exceptions to this are when there is evidence of new development of left bundle branch block or a true posterior myocardial infarction (shown by ST segment depression with dominant R waves present in leads V1 and V2). These situations require thrombolytic treatment.

Thrombolytic treatment should be given within six hours of the onset of symptoms and electrocardiographic changes for patients to derive full benefit. Patients with persisiting pain and ST segment elevation may still benefit from thrombolysis up to 12 hours from the onset of symptoms. Beyond that, few patients will benefit, and there is no clear evidence of whether this benefit outweighs the risk of haemorrhage.

Thrombolytic treatment should be offered to all eligible patients presenting with an acute myocardial infarction regardless of age, sex, or site of infarct. In general, patients over 75 years and those with anterior myocardial infarction or previous heart attack have a higher mortality. Therefore, the absolute reduction in mortality in these patients will be greater. Many of the accepted contraindications (absolute and relative) come from observational studies only. Some conditions, such as diabetic proliferative retinopathy and menstruation, are no longer considered to be absolute contraindications.

Reperfusion of the artery affected by infarction occasionally fails with thrombolytic treatment. If this happens patients will have ongoing chest pain or acute electrocardiographic changes. In these instances the optimal management is still uncertain, although readministration of an alternative thrombolytic agent ("rescue thrombolysis") or emergency percutaneous transluminal coronary angioplasty ("rescue" or "salvage" percutaneous transluminal coronary angioplasty) has been advocated. Rescue thrombolysis more than doubles the bleeding complications. Also, the limited data available showed benefit only in cases where plasma fibrinogen concentration was > 1.0 g/l and where recombinant tissue plasminogen activator was given if initial streptokinase did not achieve 25% reduction of maximal ST elevation on the pretreatment electrocardiogram.

All thrombolytic agents are plasminogen activators. Streptokinase is the cheapest widely available agent. However, it is highly antigenic, and neutralising antibodies preclude use of this agent more than once in a patient. Thus, it should not be

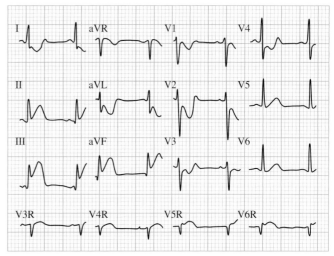

Electrocardiogram indicating acute inferior myocardial infarction

### Indications and contraindications for thrombolysis in acute myocardial infarction

#### Indications
- Clinical history and presentation strongly suggestive of myocardial infarction within 6 hours plus one or more of:
  1 mm ST elevation in two or more contiguous limb leads
  2 mm ST elevation in two or more contiguous chest leads
  New left bundle branch block
  2 mm ST depression in V1-4 suggestive of true posterior myocardial infarction
- Patients presenting with above within 7-12 hours of onset with persisting chest pains and ST segment elevation
- Patients aged < 75 years presenting within 6 hours of anterior wall myocardial infarction should be considered for recombinant tissue plasminogen activator

#### Contraindications
*Absolute*
- Aortic dissection
- Previous cerebral haemorrhage
- Known history of cerebral aneurysm or arteriovenous malformation
- Known intracranial neoplasm
- Recent (within past 6 months) thromboembolic stroke
- Active internal bleeding (excluding menstruation)
- Patients previously treated with streptokinase or anisolated plasminogen streptokinase activator complex (APSAC or anistreplase) should receive recombinant tissue plasminogen activator, reteplase, or tenecteplase

*Relative*
- Severe uncontrolled hypertension (blood pressure > 180/110 mm Hg) on presentation or chronic severe hypertension
- Current use of anticoagulants or known bleeding diathesis
- Recent (within past 2-4 weeks) trauma including head injury or traumatic or prolonged (> 10 minutes) cardiopulmonary resuscitation
- Recent (within 3 weeks) major surgery, organ biopsy, or puncture of non-compressible vessel
- Recent (within past 6 months) gastrointestinal or genitourinary or other internal bleeding
- Pregnancy
- Active peptic ulcer disease

readministered after 48 hours from the initial infusion. Tenecteplase, reteplase, and recombinant tissue plasminogen activator (alteplase) have been shown to be as good as streptokinase in reducing mortality after acute myocardial infarction. They are suitable alternatives if a patient has already received streptokinase. In the GUSTO trial, recombinant tissue plasminogen activator produced greater mortality reduction than streptokinase, especially in patients aged under 75 years who presented within six hours of onset of anterior myocardial infarction. Patients presenting within six hours of inferior myocardial infarction accompanied by right ventricular infarct, haemodynamic compromise, or anterior wall extension may also benefit. Tenecteplase has the advantage of being easily administered as a single bolus injection.

### Antiplatelet treatment

The concurrent use of aspirin with a thrombolytic drug reduces mortality far more than either drug alone. In the ISIS-2 trial, streptokinase reduced mortality by 25%, aspirin by 23%, and the combination of aspirin with streptokinase by 42%. In addition, there was no increase in incidence of stroke or major bleeding by giving aspirin and streptokinase in combination.

### Anticoagulant treatment

The use of "full dose" heparin, either intravenously or by subcutaneous injections, is not warranted routinely after streptokinase (or anistreplase) infusion, with no difference in mortality during hospitalisation and an increased risk of cerebral haemorrhage and other major bleeding. Patients who may benefit from heparin treatment after streptokinase (or anistreplase) are those at high risk of developing thromboembolism. These patients include those with large infarctions, atrial fibrillation, or congestive cardiac failure.

On the other hand, recombinant tissue plasminogen activator, tenecteplase, and reteplase have short half lives and thus have only small systemic fibrinolytic effects. The high reocclusion rates seen in patients given recombinant tissue plasminogen activator may be stopped by concomitant use of full dose heparin (for at least 24 hours). Several trials of angiographic patency have also reported a favourable synergistic effect of heparin after recombinant tissue plasminogen activator.

For patients with persistent risk factors for systemic embolisation, consideration should be given to starting oral warfarin or continuing heparin treatment as subcutaneous injections beyond 48 hours. All other patients should receive prophylactic heparin (unfractionated or low molecular weight heparin) until they are sufficiently mobile to minimise venous thromboembolism. Finally, trials comparing the use of hirudin and heparin after recombinant tissue plasminogen activator showed hirudin to be no better than heparin at reducing cardiovascular death or reinfarction at 30 days.

# Postmyocardial infarction and stable coronary artery disease

### Antiplatelet treatment

Data from the Antiplatelet Trialists' Collaboration, which analysed more than 100 trials and 100 000 patients, including 20 000 with acute myocardial infarction, confirmed that antiplatelet treatment reduced cardiovascular events in acute myocardial infarction by 25%, representing a two year treatment benefit in 36 out of 1000 patients treated.

Aspirin is the most widely used antiplatelet drug and is effective at doses from 75 to 300 mg daily in patients who have

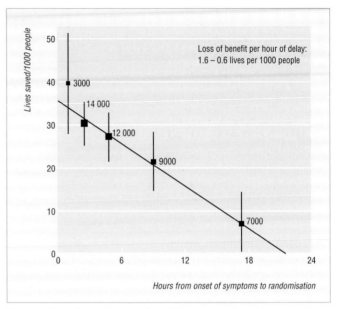

Lives saved per thousand people in relation to time of administration of thrombolytic treatment from onset of symptoms of chest pain. Numbers along the curve are the number of people treated at different times

---

**Antithrombotic therapy in acute Q wave myocardial infarction and after myocardial infarction**

**All patients should receive**
- Aspirin 300 mg orally as soon as possible and 75-300 mg daily thereafter
- Consideration for thrombolysis
- β blockers, nitrates, and other standard antianginal drugs as appropriate

**Choice of thrombolytic agents**
- Streptokinase 1.5 MU intravenously over an hour
- Recombinant tissue plasminogen activator 15 mg intravenous bolus followed by 0.75 mg/kg (maximum 50 mg) infusion over 30 minutes, then at 0.5 mg/kg (maximum 35 mg) over 60 minutes
- Reteplase 10 MU intravenous bolus, repeated once after 30 minutes
- Tenecteplase 30-50 mg (according to body weight) intravenously over 10 seconds

**Adjuvant heparin treatment**
- In all patients receiving recombinant tissue plasminogen activator— 75 U/kg intravenous bolus with recombinant tissue plasminogen activator infusion, followed by 1000-1200 U/hour to maintain APTT ratio 1.5-2.0 for 48 hours
- In all patients receiving reteplase or tenecteplase—75 U/kg intravenous bolus with first reteplase bolus, followed by 1000-1200 U/hour to maintain APTT ratio 1.5-2.0 for 48 hours

**Prevention of systemic and venous thromboembolism**
- In all patients with acute myocardial infarction—low dose low molecular weight heparin until ambulatory
- In patients receiving streptokinase at high risk of systemic or venous thromboembolism—measure APTT from four hours after thrombolysis. Start intravenous heparin at 1000-1200 U/hour once APTT ratio has fallen to less than 2.0. Continue for 48 hours, maintaining APTT at ratio 1.5-2.0. Alternatively, use low molecular weight heparin
- In all patients at high risk of systemic or venous thromboembolism—heparin infusion may be continued beyond 48 hours or converted to 15 000 U subcutaneously twice daily (alternatively, use low molecular weight heparin) or to warfarin (INR 2-3) for up to three months
- In patients with atrial fibrillation—warfarin treatment after heparin infusion should continue indefinitely

had myocardial infarction and those with stable coronary artery disease. Although there is no substantial difference in efficacy between lower and higher doses of aspirin within the stated range, higher doses are associated with greater side effects.

Dipyridamole and ticlopidine have both been compared with aspirin. Dipyridamole showed no benefit over aspirin in the PARIS trials. Ticlopidine may be slightly better than aspirin treatment but is associated with undesirable side effects such as neutropenia and thrombocytopenia. In the CAPRIE study, which compared clopidogrel with aspirin over two years in patients with vascular disease (ischaemic stroke, myocardial infarction, peripheral vascular disease), clopidogrel was slightly better in reducing the number of vascular events (5.32% $v$ 5.83%, P = 0.04). Importantly, clopidogrel was as well tolerated as aspirin. Therefore, it would be reasonable to give patients clopidogrel after acute myocardial infarction if aspirin were contraindicated or not tolerated.

The glycoprotein IIb/IIIa antagonists have been tried in conjunction with thrombolysis in acute myocardial infarction, but the various regimens used in recent trials did not confer any additional benefit over conventional treatment. However, there was some evidence of more rapid and complete reperfusion, and these agents warrant further evaluation and refinement.

### Anticoagulant treatment

Long term anticoagulation with heparin followed by warfarin is not needed routinely except in patients at higher risk of venous or systemic thromboembolism.

Intracardiac thrombi usually occur within 48 hours after acute myocardial infarction and tend to embolise within the first few weeks. Low dose dalteparin has been shown to reduce the incidence of intramural thrombus (21.9% $v$ 14.2%, P = 0.03) in patients given thrombolytic treatments, although this is at a risk of small increase in minor bleeding complications. Thus, in patients at high risk of mural thrombus formation, dalteparin should be started as soon as possible after the diagnosis of acute myocardial infarction.

Warfarin should be continued for two to three months, except in the case of atrial fibrillation, when it may be maintained indefinitely. While a patient is taking warfarin, aspirin use may increase the risk of bleeding, but, pending further evidence, many clinicians still continue to use low dose aspirin for its antiplatelet effect. Although thrombus is commonly associated with left ventricular aneurysm (up to 60%), systemic emboli are uncommon (4-5%), and long term anticoagulation does not seem to further reduce the risk of systemic embolisation; thus, anticoagulant treatment is not currently indicated in these patients in the long term.

Venous thromboembolism is often associated with acute myocardial infarction, although its incidence has fallen since the introduction of thrombolytic treatment. Although no trials have compared the efficacy of low molecular weight heparin with unfractionated heparin in preventing venous thromboembolism after acute myocardial infarction per se, it is likely that these agents are equally effective, and are increasingly used in clinical practice.

The box showing antithrombotic therapy in acute Q wave myocardial infarction and after myocardial infarction is adapted from the 6th ACCP consensus conference on antithrombotic therapy. The figure showing lives saved in relation to time of administration of thrombolytic treatment from onset of symptoms of chest pain is adapted from Collins R, et al, *N Engl J Med* 1997;336:847-60.

### Risk factors for systemic embolisation when anticoagulation should be considered

- Large anterior wall myocardial infarction
- Myocardial infarction complicated by severe left ventricular dysfunction
- Congestive heart failure
- Echocardiographic evidence of mural thrombus or left ventricular aneurysm
- Previous emboli
- Atrial fibrillation

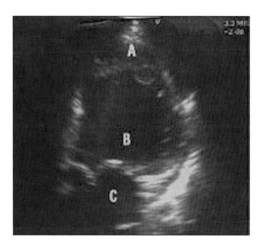

Echocardiogram showing thrombus at left ventricular apex in patient with dilated cardiomyopathy (A=thrombus, B=left ventricle, C=left atrium)

### Further reading

- Cairns JA, Theroux P, Lewis D, Ezekowitz M, Meade TW. Antithrombotic agents in coronary artery disease. *Chest* 2001;119:228–52S
- Collins R, MacMahon S, Flather M, Baigent C, Remvig L, Mortensen S, et al. Clinical effects of anticoagulant therapy in suspected acute myocardial infarction: systematic overview of randomised trials. *BMJ* 1996;313:652-9
- ISIS-2 Collaborative Group. Randomised trial of intravenous streptokinase, oral aspirin, both, or neither among 17,187 cases of suspected acute myocardial infarction: ISIS-2. *Lancet* 1988;II:349-60
- Oldroyd KG. Identifying failure to achieve complete (TIMI 3) reperfusion following thrombolytic treatment: how to do it, when to do it, and why it's worth doing. *Heart* 2000;84:113-5
- Mounsey JP, Skinner JS, Hawkins T, MacDermott AF, Furniss SS, Adams PC, et al. Rescue thrombolysis: alteplase as adjuvant treatment after streptokinase in acute myocardial infarction. *Br Heart J* 1995;74:348-53
- The GUSTO Investigators. An international randomized trial comparing 4 thrombolytic strategies for acute myocardial infarction. *N Eng J Med* 1993;329:673-82
- National Institute for Clinical Excellence. *Technology appraisal guideline no 52. Guidance on the use of drugs for early thrombolysis in the treatment of acute myocaardial infarction.* London: NICE, 2002
- Ohman EM, Harrington RA, Cannon CP, Agnelli G, Cairns JA, Kennedy JW. Intravenous thrombolysis in acute myocardial infarction. *Chest* 2001;119:253-77S

# 11 Antithrombotic therapy in acute coronary syndromes

Robert D S Watson, Bernard S P Chin, Gregory Y H Lip

The use of antithrombotic therapy in acute coronary syndromes has reduced the incidence of death and Q wave myocardial infarction dramatically in recent years. Antithrombotic drugs in routine use include antiplatelet drugs (aspirin, clopidogrel, and glycoprotein IIb/IIIa receptor antagonists) and anticoagulants (unfractionated and low molecular weight heparin, warfarin, and direct thrombin inhibitors).

## Pathogenesis

Thrombosis is the basic pathophysiological process underlying the acute coronary syndromes. Thus, antithrombotic therapy is the cornerstone of management, and the appropriate choice of antithrombotic drugs to reduce platelet aggregation or interfere with the clotting process can be critical.

Rupture of the fibrous cap of an atheromatous plaque exposes the lipid core, which is highly thrombogenic and contains an abundance of procoagulant tissue factor. Plaque rupture (exposing surface binding glycoproteins) allows platelets to adhere to the plaque, become activated, and release thromboxane A2, which causes further platelet aggregation and vasoconstriction. As the platelets aggregate around the ruptured plaque, membrane glycoprotein IIb/IIIa receptors undergo a configuration change to bind fibrinogen and form a complex platelet linkage. Further incorporation of fibrin and red blood cells within this platelet-rich thrombus results in a partial or total occlusion of the coronary artery. Alternatively, thrombus may break off from a ruptured plaque and occlude a downstream vessel. Occlusion may also follow from trapping of circulating thrombi formed elsewhere in the circulation.

## Antithrombotic drugs

### Antiplatelet drugs

*Aspirin*

Aspirin has been in use for more than 150 years and is cheap and effective. It has been shown to reduce the risk of fatal and non-fatal myocardial infarction by at least 50% in patients with unstable angina. Aspirin blocks cyclo-oxygenase and formation of thromboxane A2, thus reducing platelet aggregation induced via this pathway.

Aspirin is the cornerstone of treatment in acute coronary syndromes and chronic coronary artery disease. The beneficial effects of aspirin seem to be sustained for at least two years and regardless of the dose used. However, 75-150 mg daily may have a lower incidence of gastrointestinal side effects than the higher doses used in some randomised studies.

*ADP receptor antagonists*

Ticlopidine and clopidogrel are ADP inhibitors. Evidence exists that ticlopidine reduces mortality, recurrent infarction, stroke, and angina at least to six months after myocardial infarction or unstable angina. Ticlodipine has fewer gastrointestinal effects than aspirin but may cause reversible neutropenia and thrombocytopenia ($< 1\%$ of patients), which dictates therapeutic monitoring with regular blood counts.

Clopidogrel is a derivative of ticlopidine that seems to be six times more effective than its predecessor in preventing platelet

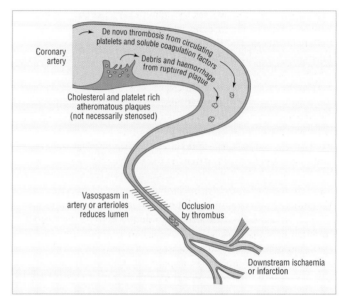

Thrombosis in relation to acute coronary syndromes

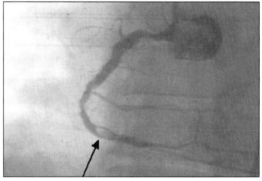

Thrombus within right coronary artery (arrow) in a patient with unstable angina

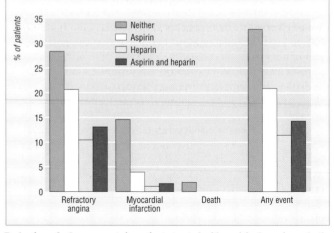

Reduction of adverse events in patients treated with aspirin, heparin, or both compared with neither drug

aggregation. Clopidogrel has shown better tolerability with less bleeding than aspirin and fewer haematological side effects than ticlopidine. In the CURE trial—a randomised, double blind, parallel group study of 12 562 patients with acute coronary syndrome or non-Q wave myocardial infarction—patients received aspirin 75-325 mg and then were randomly assigned to additional clopidogrel (300 mg load followed by 75 mg daily) or placebo for three months to a year. Additional clopidogrel resulted in a 20% relative risk reduction in the primary end point (cardiovascular death, myocardial infarction, or stroke) (P < 0.0001), mainly caused by a 23% relative reduction in myocardial infarction. However, there was a 34% excess of major bleeding (3.6% v 2.7% in placebo; P = 0.003).

These observations raise the question of whether combination antiplatelet treatment (such as aspirin with clopidogrel) is preferable to other treatments (such as heparin with glycoprotein IIb/IIIa receptor inhibitors) in the acute phase of acute coronary syndromes and suggest that prolonged antiplatelet treatment is better for high risk patients.

*Glycoprotein IIb/IIIa receptor inhibitors*
Abciximab is a (large molecule) monoclonal antibody and the first glycoprotein IIb/IIIa receptor antagonist to be developed. Eptifibatide is a peptide receptor antagonist, whereas tirofiban is a non-peptide receptor antagonist. Both eptifibatide and tirofiban are small molecules, apparently non-immunogenic, and therefore suitable for repeat infusions. They have a shorter half life (90-120 minutes) than abciximab (12 hours). Because they are mainly renally cleared, their doses should be adjusted in patients with renal impairment.

In trials with patients with acute coronary syndromes the rate of death, reinfarction, and refractory angina was reduced when glycoprotein IIb/IIIa inhibitors were added to aspirin and heparin. In the largest study, PURSUIT, a bolus injection of eptifibatide followed by a 72 hour infusion resulted in a 9.6% relative risk reduction in death and myocardial infarction when given to patients with acute coronary syndromes already receiving aspirin and heparin. In the PRISM and PRISM-PLUS studies, tirofiban, when given in addition to aspirin and heparin, achieved a 43% relative risk reduction in mortality and reinfarction at seven days. This benefit was sustained at 30 days. Patients taking tirofiban and aspirin without heparin had an excess mortality rate, and this treatment arm was stopped early.

The CAPTURE trial studied patients with acute coronary syndromes scheduled for percutaneous coronary angioplasty. The use of abciximab for about 24 hours before the procedure substantially reduced the risk of mortality, myocardial infarction, or need to proceed to other revascularisation.

The benefits are greatest in patients with elevated levels of troponin T or I, indicating that assessment of subtle indices of cardiac damage predicts patients at higher risk and those most likely to benefit from treatment. Economic evaluations of the costs of using intravenous glycoprotein IIb/IIIa inhibitors suggest that, for patients with elevated troponin levels, 11 are needed to be treated to prevent one death or acute myocardial infarction at 30 days. The equivalent cost effectiveness is about £5000 an outcome.

Using glycoprotein IIb/IIIa inhibitors for acute coronary syndrome in addition to conventional antithrombotic therapy is approved by the British National Institute for Clinical Excellence (NICE). However, interpretation of trial evidence is complicated by patient heterogeneity. Although adjunctive treatment before revascularisation procedures in acute coronary syndromes shows clear benefit, there is some uncertainty of benefit if these drugs are used only as "medical" management without revascularisation.

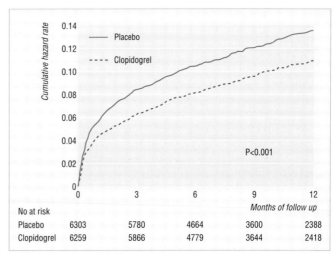

Effects of clopidogrel plus aspirin in patients with acute coronary syndromes without ST segment elevation. From the clopidogrel in unstable angina to prevent recurrent events (CURE) trial investigators

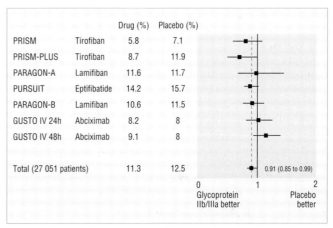

Glycoprotein IIb/IIIa inhibitors v conventional treatment in six trials. Results show odds ratio (95% confidence interval) for death and myocardial infarction at 30 day follow up

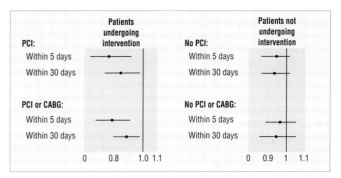

Glycoprotein IIb/IIIa inhibitors in patients with acute coronary syndromes: patients undergoing percutaneous coronary intervention and patients not undergoing percutaneous coronary intervention. Results show odds ratio (95% confidence interval) for death or myocardial infarction (CABG=coronary artery bypass graft surgery, PCI=percutaneous coronary intervention)

## Anticoagulant treatment

### Low molecular weight heparin

Low molecular weight heparins possess more anti-Xa activity than unfractionated heparins. They have a more predictable anticoagulant effect and cause less thrombocytopenia. Titrated appropriately against body weight, low molecular weight heparin provides effective anticoagulation and does not need regular monitoring of the activated partial thromboplastin time. However, platelet count monitoring to detect thrombocytopenia is recommended if treatment is extended beyond a few days. Studies suggest similar safety profiles to unfractionated heparin when used with glycoprotein IIb/IIIa inhibitors.

The therapeutic benefits of low molecular weight heparins are now clear. Recent randomised trials comparing the efficacy of various low molecular weight heparins showed enoxaparin and nadroparin to be more effective in reducing mortality in unstable angina than either aspirin or unfractionated heparin alone. In the ESSENCE study, enoxaparin reduced the incidence of death, myocardial infarction, and reccurent angina at 14 days from 19.6% to 16.6% when compared with unfractionated heparin. This benefit was maintained at 30 days and a year.

Dalteparin in addition to aspirin was more effective than aspirin alone in the FRISC study. It reduced cardiac events and death (1.8% v 4.8%) when used in acute coronary syndromes but was no better than adjusted dose unfractionated heparin.

Low molecular weight heparin is, therefore, at least as good as unfractionated heparin in managing unstable angina (with trials showing enoxaparin and nadroparin to be even better). It has practical advantages because it has more consistent antithrombin effects and is easier to administer, and frequent assessment of antithrombotic effect (activated partial thromboplastin time monitoring) is not neccesary. In view of these findings, low molecular weight heparins (enoxaparin and nadroparin) should be used routinely to treat unstable angina concurrently with aspirin in place of unfractionated heparin.

### Unfractionated heparin

An uncontrolled study showed that heparin treatment in unstable angina reduced the risk of progression to myocardial infarction by 80%. Other studies show a definite reduction in the incidence of refractory angina and myocardial infarction with the use of unfractionated heparin compared with placebo (risk reduction 0.29). Treatment with heparin and aspirin seems to be more effective than either heparin or aspirin alone. In a meta-analysis on the effect of adding heparin to aspirin in patients with unstable angina, combination treatment resulted in 33% reduction in deaths or myocardial infarction.

### Direct thrombin inhibitors

Newer and powerful anticoagulants, such as the direct thrombin inhibitor hirudin, are being investigated. Several trials compared the effects of hirudin with unfractionated heparin and showed a slight reduction in primary end points, and a pooled analysis of these trials showed a 22% relative risk reduction in myocardial infarction or deaths at 72 hours. Bleeding, however, may be a problem. Hirudin is now approved for patients with heparin induced thrombocytopenia but is not yet licensed for treatment of acute coronary syndromes. The direct thrombin inhibitors melagatran and ximelagatran are currently under investigation for use in patients with acute coronary syndromes.

### Warfarin

Several trials have investigated using warfarin for unstable angina. In many studies, warfarin was given to patients two days after unfractionated heparin infusion and continued for ten weeks to six months with an international normalised ratio (INR) adjusted

---

**Antithrombotic therapy is the cornerstone of management in acute coronary syndromes**

| Trial | LMWH | Timing of endpoint | Event rate (%) LMWH | Event rate (%) UH |
|---|---|---|---|---|
| **Short term results:** | | | | |
| FRIC | Dalteparin | Day 1-6 | 3.9 | 3.6 |
| ESSENCE | Enoxaparin | Day 14 | 4.6 | 6.1 |
| TIMI 11-B | Enoxaparin | Day 14 | 5.7 | 6.9 |
| FRAXIS | Nadroparin | Day 14 | 4.9 | 4.5 |
| Total | | | | 0.86 (0.72 to 1.02) P=0.07 |
| **Long term results:** | | | | |
| FRIC | Dalteparin | Day 6-45 | 4.3 | 4.7 |
| ESSENCE | Enoxaparin | Day 43 | 6.2 | 8.2 |
| TIMI 11-B | Enoxaparin | Day 43 | 7.9 | 8.9 |
| FRAXIS | Nadroparin | Day 90 | 8.9 | 7.9 |
| Total | | | | 0.89 (0.77 to 1.03) P=0.12 |

Comparison of low molecular weight heparins with unfractionated heparins in patients with acute coronary syndromes. Results show odds ratio (95% confidence interval) for death and myocardial infarction at long and short term follow up (LMWH=low molecular weight heparin, UH=unfractionated heparin)

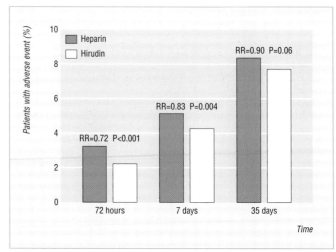

Comparison of hirudin therapy with unfractionated heparin in patients with acute coronary syndromes (RR=relative risk)

to between 2.0 and 3.0. Earlier studies showed low fixed doses of warfarin gave no benefit. However, limited evidence suggests that in patients with acute coronary syndromes, combination treatment with aspirin and warfarin adjusted to INR 2.0-3.0 may reduce event rates and hospitalisations.

Pending further trials and in view of potential bleeding risks and need for INR monitoring, warfarin is best reserved for patients with other indications for warfarin use such as coexistent atrial fibrillation, known left ventricular aneurysm with mural thrombus formation, or previous recurrent thromboembolic stroke. Warfarin should not be used as the sole antithrombotic drug in acute cases because of its delayed onset of action.

# Thrombolytic treatment

Thrombolytic treatment is not recommended for unstable angina and non-Q wave infarction. It has not been shown to reduce cardiovascular events and death and may worsen clinical outcomes by increasing bleeding complications, as well as increasing bleeding within a ruptured atherosclerotic plaque. This worsens obstruction to coronary flow and exposes clot-bound thrombin to flowing blood, creating an even more prothrombotic environment. In addition, the thrombus in unstable angina is often platelet-rich, unlike the fibrin-rich thrombus seen in infarction, and thus may be less responsive to thrombolytic treatment.

The figure showing reduction of adverse events in patients treated with aspirin, heparin sodium, or both compared with neither drug is adapted from Theroux P et al, *N Engl J Med* 1988;319;1105-11. The effects of clopidogrel plus aspirin in patients with acute coronary syndromes is adapted from the CURE trial investigators, *N Engl J Med* 2001;345: 494-502. The figures showing glycoprotein IIb/IIIa inhibitors *v* conventional treatment, comparing the effects glycoprotein IIb/IIIa inhibitors in acute coronary syndrome patients who are undergoing percutaneous coronary intervention with those who are not, and comparing low molecular weight heparin with unfractionated heparin in patients with acute coronary syndrome are all adapted from Bertrand M, et al, *Eur Heart J* 2002;23:1809-40. The figure comparing hirudin treatment with unfractionated heparin in patients with acute coronary syndromes is adapted from Glenn N et al, *Arch Intern Med* 2001;161:937-48

## Antithrombotic therapy in acute coronary syndromes: a summary

### Aspirin
- Acute treatment with aspirin is used in all patients with suspected acute coronary syndromes in the absence of contraindications and for long term treatment thereafter

### Clopidogrel
- In acute coronary syndrome patients clopidogrel is used for acute treatment and for longer term treatment for at least 9-12 months. Beyond this, treatment will depend on the risk status of the patient and individual clinical judgment
- Clopidogrel is used for immediate and long term treatment in patients who do not tolerate aspirin and in patients receiving a stent
- Clopidogrel is given to acute coronary syndrome patients scheduled for angiography unless there is a likelihood that the patient will proceed to urgent surgery (within 5 days)

### Low molecular weight heparin
- In aspirin treated patients, low molecular weight heparin is better than placebo. There are also data in favour of low molecular weight heparin (enoxaparin) over unfractionated heparin when administered as an acute regimen

### Glycoprotein IIb/IIIa receptor inhibitors
- Treatment with a glycoprotein IIb/IIIa receptor blocker is recommended in all patients with acute coronary syndromes undergoing percutaneous coronary interventions. The infusion should be continued for 12 hours (abciximab) or 24 hours (eptifibatide, tirofiban) after the procedure
- Medical treatment with a glycoprotein IIb/IIIa receptor blocker during the first days after admission, followed by percutaneous coronary intervention or bypass surgery, yields a significant reduction in death and non-fatal myocardial infarction at 72 hours, from 4.3 to 2.9%
- Diabetic patients with acute coronary syndrome derive particular benefit from glycoprotein IIb/IIIa receptor inhibitors

### Fibrinolytic treatment
- In contrast to acute coronary syndromes *with* ST segment elevation, thrombolytic therapy is not recommended for patients with acute coronary syndromes *without* persistent ST segment elevation

## Further reading

- Anand SS, Yusuf S, Pogue J, Weitz JI, Flather M. Long term oral anticoagulant therapy in patients with unstable angina or suspected non-Q wave myocardial infarction. The OASIS (warfarin) substudy. *Circulation* 1998;98:1064-70
- British Cardiac Society Guidelines and Medical Practice Committee, and Royal College of Physicians Clinical Effectiveness and Evaluation Unit. Guideline for the management of patients with acute coronary syndrome without persistent ECG ST segment elevation. *Heart* 2001;85:133-42
- The CAPTURE Investigators. Randomised placebo controlled trial of abciximab before and during intervention in refractory unstable angina: The CAPTURE study. *Lancet* 1997;349:1429-35
- Cohen M, Demers C, Gurfinkel EP, Turpie AG, Fromell GJ, Goodman S, et al. A comparison of low molecular weight heparin with unfractionated heparin for unstable coronary artery disease (ESSENCE). *N Engl J Med* 1997;337:447-52
- Fragmin and fast revascularisation during instability in coronary artery disease (FRISC-II) Investigators. Long term low molecular mass heparin in unstable coronary artery disease: FRISC-II prospective multicentre randomised study. *Lancet* 1999;354:701-7
- PRISM-PLUS Investigators. Inhibiton of the platelet glycoprotein IIb/IIIa receptor with tirofiban in unstable angina and non Q-wave myocardial infarction. *N Engl J Med* 1998;338:1488-97
- The PURSUIT Trial Investigators. Inhibiton of platelet glycoprotein IIb/IIIa with eptifibatide in patients with acute coronary syndromes. *N Engl J Med* 1998;339:436-43
- National Institute for Clinical Excellence (NICE). Guidance on the use of glycoprotein IIb/IIIa inhibitors in the treatment of acute coronary syndromes. NICE Technology Appraisal Guidance No 12. London: NICE, 2000
- Task force on the management of acute coronary syndromes of the European Society of Cardiology. Management of acute coronary syndromes in patients presenting without persistent ST-segment elevation. *Eur Heart J* 2002;23:1809-40

# 12 Antithrombotic strategies in acute coronary syndromes and percutaneous coronary interventions

Derek L Connolly, Gregory Y H Lip, Bernard S P Chin

## Acute coronary syndromes

All patients suspected of having acute coronary syndrome should be managed as medical emergencies and monitored in the critical care unit. Baseline tests must include 12 lead electrocardiography, chest x ray examination, and venous blood samples for analyses of haemoglobin and markers of myocardial damage, preferably cardiac troponin T or I.

### Initial management

*Assessment*

Patients with persistent ST segment elevation on 12 lead electrocardiography need immediate reperfusion treatment (thrombolysis or intervention). Patients with ST segment depression, inverted T waves, or pseudonormalisation of T waves on the electrocardiogram, but with a clinical history suggesting cardiac ischaemia should receive initial treatment for angina.

This would include aspirin 300 mg followed by a low dose of 75-150 mg daily. In cases of aspirin intolerance, clopidogrel should be used. β Blockers and nitrates should also be given. Rate limiting calcium antagonists can be used if β blockers are contraindicated or are already being used. Ideally, patients should be given low molecular weight heparin (such as enoxaparin) according to their weight. If low molecular weight heparin is unavailable, unfractionated heparin may be used. A bolus of 5000 U is given, followed by an infusion adjusted to get an activated partial thromboplastin time (APTT) ratio of 1.8 to 2.5. In light of data from the CURE and PCI-CURE study, clopidogrel (given for at least one month and up to nine months) should be considered in addition to aspirin when an early non-interventional approach is planned. The optimal dose of aspirin to limit bleeding is probably 75 mg, particularly with clopidogrel. A glycoprotein IIb/IIIa receptor inhibitor should be added to aspirin and heparin for patients in whom catheterisation and percutaneous coronary intervention are planned. In these patients clopidogrel could be considered if they are not at high risk for bleeding.

*Observation*

Patients should be observed over the next eight to 12 hours. Patients at high risk of progressing to acute myocardial infarction or death should receive a glycoprotein IIb/IIIa receptor inhibitor (eptifibatide or tirofiban) in addition to heparin and aspirin or clopidogrel (alone or with asprin). Abciximab would be used in high risk patients undergoing percutaneous coronary intervention. There is no role for thrombolytic therapy in patients without acute ST segment elevation, except in the situations of a true posterior myocardial infarction, or a presumed new left bundle branch block.

### Subsequent management

When patients have been free from symptoms and ischaemic electrocardiographic changes for >48 hours, and any intravenous treatments and heparin have been stopped for >24 hours, risk assessment with stress testing should be performed unless contraindicated. Stress testing for risk assessment is unnecessary if a patient is already in a high risk category for which coronary angiography is indicated.

---

**High and low risk patients with suspected acute coronary syndromes**

**High risk**
- Recurrent or persistent chest pains with associated electrocardiographic changes (ST segment depression or transient ST elevation) despite anti-ischaemic treatment
- Elevated troponin concentrations
- Age >65 years
- Comorbidity, especially diabetes
- Development of pulmonary oedema or haemodynamic instability within observation period
- Development of major arrhythmias (repetitive ventricular tachycardia or ventricular fibrillation)
- Early postinfarction unstable angina

**Low risk**
- No recurrence of chest pains within observation period
- Troponin or other markers of myocardial damage not elevated
- No ST segment depression or elevation on electrocardiogram (T wave inversion is classified as intermediate risk)

---

**Management strategies for patients with suspected acute coronary syndromes, with risk stratification by troponin and stress tests***

**Low risk**
*Results of tests*
- Cardiac troponin result is negative or low (troponin T <0.01 µg/l or troponin I equivalent) on two occasions
- Stress test indicates a low risk category

*Action*
- If free from cardiac symptoms, no more cardiac interventions needed
- Subsequent outpatient review appropriate for further investigations and adjustment of drug treatment

**Intermediate risk**
*Results of tests*
- Impaired left ventricular function, or haemodynamic abnormalities or arrhythmia during the acute phase *but*
- Normal cardiac troponin result (troponin T <0.01 µg/l, or troponin I equivalent), with a stress test indicating intermediate risk *or*
- Moderately elevated cardiac troponin (troponin T 0.01-0.1 µg/l, or troponin I equivalent) with stress test indicating low risk category

*Action*
- Many cardiologists perform coronary angiography on these patients, but clear evidence of benefit is lacking

**High risk**
*Results of tests*
- Maximal cardiac troponin result is high (troponin T >0.1 µg/l, or troponin I equivalent) *or*
- Stress test indicates high risk category

*Action*
- Coronary angiography should be arranged, unless contraindicated, and performed urgently, before discharge from hospital
- Patients with suitable lesions for percutaneous coronary intervention should be given clopidogrel, which should also be given to patients with coronary lesions not suitable for any revascularisation

*If patient is unable to perform an exercise electrocardiogram, an alternative non-exercise (pharmacological) stress test, such as a stress echocardiograph or isotope myocardial stress perfusion study, should be arranged unless contraindicated. In all cases, aggressive risk factor management and regular aspirin treatment (or clopidogrel, or both, depending on clinical situation) is necessary

*Antithrombotic treatment*

Low molecular weight heparin should be given for at least two days, and for up to eight days or longer in cases of recurrent ischaemia or where myocardial revascularisation is delayed or contraindicated. Patients requiring a bypass operation may have their glycoprotein IIb/IIIa receptor antagonist infusion stopped before or at the time of cardiac surgery, although clopidogrel should be withheld for five to seven days.

## Risk stratification and antithrombotic strategies

Recent trials have shown that patients with elevated troponin benefit from treatment with low molecular weight heparin, glycoprotein IIb/IIIa blockers, or an invasive strategy, whereas patients without troponin elevation showed no such benefit.

In these high risk patients, angiography with a view to revascularisation should be performed on the same admission. Infusion of glycoprotein IIb/IIIa receptor inhibitors should be started while waiting and preparing for angiography and continued for 12 hours (abciximab) or 24 hours (tirofiban) after angioplasty is performed.

Low risk patients can be mobilised and discharged if (at least 12 hours after the onset of symptoms of a suspected acute coronary syndrome) the symptoms have not recurred, cardiac troponin concentrations are normal, electrocardiograms remain normal (or unchanged compared with a recording from before the current presentation), and cardiac enzyme activities are not raised. Risk assessment with stress testing should be performed before a patient is discharged unless contraindicated.

## Pros and cons of invasive strategy

There are arguments for and against an invasive approach to acute coronary syndromes. In the FRISC-II trial an invasive strategy had, after a year, saved 1.7 lives in 100 patients and prevented 2.0 non-fatal myocardial infarctions and 20 readmissions. It provided earlier and better symptom relief at the cost of 15 more patients with coronary artery bypass grafting and 21 more with percutaneous transluminal coronary angioplasty, and these results were independent of treatment with dalteparin or placebo. In the BHF RITA3 trial of patients with unstable angina, myocardial infarction, or non-ST segment elevation, an invasive strategy reduced refractory or severe angina, with no increase of death or myocardial infarction, compared with a conservative strategy. Against these benefits is the need to have adequate provision of facilities and trained staff to undertake such procedures.

# Percutaneous coronary intervention

Arterial thrombi occur soon after percutaneous coronary interventions for coronary artery disease, usually at the site of the dilated segment. Arterial thrombi are rich in platelets, red blood cells, fibrin, and leucocytes and may contribute to vessel reocclusion with the consequent need for revascularisation. The risk of reocclusion depends on the extent of segment dilatation and vessel injury, as well as local shear forces. Antiplatelet and antithrombin drugs generally reduce the risk of occlusion or the need for further intervention but are not perfect. Where facilities are available, percutaneous coronary angioplasty is an alternative to thrombolytic treatment as a means of reperfusion in acute myocardial infarction.

## Antiplatelet treatment

Patients with coronary artery disease undergoing angioplasty should continue taking antiplatelet drugs as usual. For patients not receiving regular antiplatelet treatment, aspirin 100-325 mg should be given orally at least two hours before angioplasty.

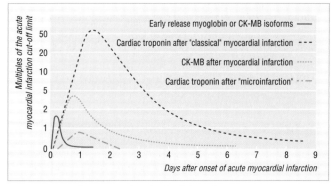

Time course of different cardiac biochemical markers

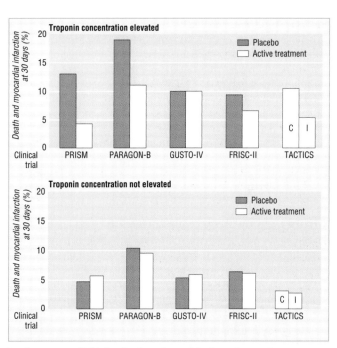

Death or myocardial infarction in patients with elevated troponin concentration or negative troponin result in contemporary trials. The FRISC-II trial also used low molecular weight heparin, and the bars for the TACTICS trial show the strategies used (I=invasive strategy, C=conservative strategy)

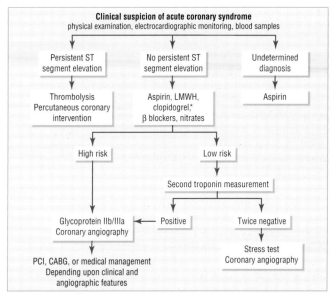

European Society of Cardiology recommended strategy for acute coronary syndromes (CABG=coronary artery bypass graft, LMWH=low molecular weight heparin, PCI=percutaneous coronary intervention. *Omit clopidogrel if patient likely to go to CABG within 5 days)

Aspirin substantially reduces the rate of intracoronary thrombus formation at the treatment site and restenoses. The addition of dipyridamole to aspirin adds little extra benefit and is not recommended. Ticlopidine alone has not been shown to be more effective than aspirin alone in patients undergoing percutaneous interventions. Although clopidogrel is marginally better than aspirin in patients with atherosclerotic vascular disease (CAPRIE study), direct comparisons between aspirin and clopidogrel in coronary intervention have not revealed marked differences. Thus, ticlopidine and clopidogrel are useful alternatives for patients scheduled for percutaneous coronary angioplasty who are unable to take aspirin.

After intervention, antiplatelet combination treatment (aspirin plus ticlopidine) is superior to aspirin alone at reducing ischaemic complications and cardiac events, particularly after intracoronary stent placements. The stent anticoagulation restenosis investigators (SARI) trial, compared aspirin-ticlopidine combination treatment with aspirin-warfarin combination treatment and aspirin alone and showed that patients taking aspirin-ticlopidine had the best 30 day mortality (0.5% $v$ 2.7% $v$ 3.6% respectively, P = 0.001). Total bleeding complications occurred in 5.5% of those taking aspirin-ticlopidine, quite high when compared with 1.8% in those taking aspirin only (P < 0.001), and the incidence of neutropenia was not significantly different. The CLASSICS trial showed clopidogrel-aspirin combination treatment to be as effective as ticlopidine-aspirin combination treatment after angioplasty and stent placement.

### Glycoprotein IIb/IIIa receptor antagonists

Despite adequate treatment with antiplatelet drugs, platelet activation still continues along other pathways not blocked by these agents. This is where the glycoprotein IIb/IIIa receptor antagonists, which block the final common pathways of platelet aggregation, have contributed most to the management of angioplasty and stenting.

Abciximab, eptifibatide, and tirofiban have all been shown to reduce reocclusion and cardiovascular events, including deaths and myocardial infarctions, at 30 days when used in patients undergoing elective and urgent angioplasty and stenting. These benefits are additional to those achieved with antiplatelet drugs, and the effects were most prominent with abciximab. The EPIC, EPILOG, and CAPTURE trials all showed that abciximab infusion reduced major complication rates during balloon angioplasty, a benefit that was sustained at 30 days' follow up. The EPISTENT trial showed that abciximab reduces major complications during stent placement and was superior to a combination of abciximab and balloon angioplasty. In the only direct comparison of glycoprotein IIb/IIIa antagonists, the TARGET trial randomised 5308 patients to tirofiban or abciximab before percutaneous transluminal coronary angioplasty or stent, or both: by six months the primary end point was similar in both treatment arms (14.9% with tirofiban $v$ 14.3% with abciximab, P > 0.05), as was mortality (1.9% $v$ 1.7%, P > 0.05). Patients with unstable angina, acute myocardial infarction, and other risk factors (such as diabetes) for postprocedure in stent thrombosis or restenosis stand to benefit most from glycoprotein IIb/IIIa receptor antagonists.

In light of this, glycoprotien IIb/IIIa drugs should be considered in all patients at risk of developing in stent stenosis or with acute coronary syndrome scheduled for percutaneous coronary interventions. If percutaneous coronary intervention is planned in unstable angina, glycoprotein IIb/IIIa receptor antagonist infusions should be started before intervention and continued for 12 hours (abciximab) or 24 hours (tirofiban, eptifibatide) after the procedure.

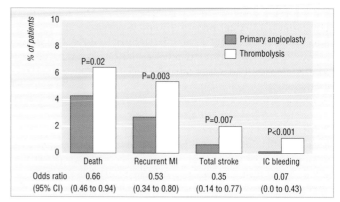

| Odds ratio (95% CI) | Death 0.66 (0.46 to 0.94) | Recurrent MI 0.53 (0.34 to 0.80) | Total stroke 0.35 (0.14 to 0.77) | IC bleeding 0.07 (0.0 to 0.43) |
|---|---|---|---|---|

Meta-analysis of 10 randomised trials that compared thrombolytic treatment with primary angioplasty in acute myocardial infarction (MI=myocardial infarction, IC=intracranial)

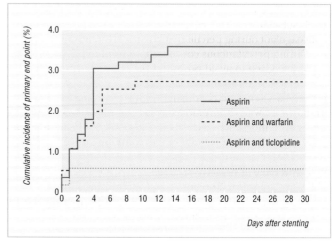

Cumulative incidence of primary end points (mortality, target lesion revascularisation or thrombosis, non-fatal myocardial infarction) in patients treated with aspirin alone (557 patients), aspirin and warfarin (550 patients), or aspirin and ticlopidine (546 patients) after coronary artery stenting

---

**Some factors predisposing to in stent thrombosis after placement**

- Underdilation of the stent
- Proximal and distal dissections
- Vessel diameter < 3 mm
- Poor inflow
- Outflow obstruction

---

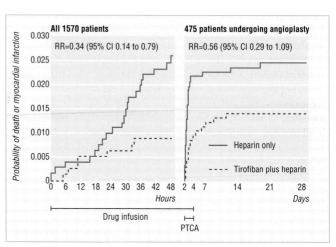

PRISM-PLUS results showing cumulative incidence of death or myocardial infarction (PTCA=percutaneous transluminal coronary angioplasty, RR=relative risk)

Several economic evaluations have found that routine use of glycoprotein IIb/IIIa drugs after percutaneous coronary interventions is extremely cost effective for patients at high risk of myocardial infarction or death. In such patients, the number needed to treat to save one life or prevent one acute myocardial infarction at 30 days may be as low as 30, or about £5000 per outcome.

## Anticoagulant treatment

Most patients with acute coronary syndromes undergoing angioplasty would have been pretreated with heparin. Several small studies have shown that patients with unstable angina who receive heparin before intervention have a higher rate of success and lower postprocedure reocclusion rates.

Increasing numbers of patients with unstable angina are now being treated with low molecular weight heparin. However, such drugs tend to have a longer half life than unfractionated heparin and their effects are not completely reversed by protamine sulphate if necessary. Low molecular weight heparins can be safely substituted for unfractionated heparin as a procedural anticoagulant during percutaneous coronary intervention.

During percutaneous coronary interventions, heparin should be given to avoid postprocedure complications. The dose of unfractionated heparin given should be sufficient to increase the activated clotting time (ACT) to 250-300 seconds as measured with the HemoTec device (or 300-350 seconds with the Hemochron device). Unfractionated heparin dose may need to be adjusted for weight or sex. If glycoprotein IIb/IIIa receptor agonists are being used, then unfractionated heparin boluses should be reduced to achieve a target ACT of about 200 seconds. Although the traditional means of assessing heparin anticoagulation has been with the APTT, the ACT is an assay of whole blood clotting time that can be performed rapidly at the bedside and catheterisation laboratory.

Routine use of unfractionated heparin (either as infusion or subcutaneously) after angioplasty is probably not indicated for uncomplicated procedures. Studies have shown excess bleeding complications with heparin treatment without a reduction in the number of cardiac ischaemic events. Patients who do not receive heparin treatment after coronary interventions can have their femoral sheaths removed earlier, resulting in shorter hospital stays, fewer bleeding complications, at the risk of a similar incidence of cardiac end points including reocclusion.

With the advent of glycoprotein IIb/IIIa receptor antagonists, heparin infusions postprocedure should not be necessary routinely. Femoral sheaths should be removed once the ACT has fallen to less than 150-180 seconds. Adjunctive treatment with low molecular weight heparin or unfractionated heparin may still be warranted after angioplasty and stent implantation in patients at high risk of in stent thrombosis.

Full anticoagulation with heparin followed by warfarin in patients undergoing angioplasty with stenting is no better at reducing the number of adverse effects than combination treatment with aspirin and ticlopidine, but at increased risk of bleeding with warfarin. Use of hirudin, the direct thrombin inhibitor, was associated with a reduction of early cardiac events and restenosis at 96 hours but was no different from the heparin treatment arm at seven months.

## Antithrombotic therapy in coronary angioplasty and stent placement procedures

### Before procedure
- Aspirin 80-325 mg once daily at least 2 hours before procedure. Ticlopidine 250 mg twice daily or clopidogrel 75 mg once daily started 24 hours before procedure if aspirin contraindicated
- Glycoprotein IIb/IIIa receptor antagonists should be considered in high risk patients with acute coronary syndromes

### During and after procedure
- Heparin* bolus to achieve activated clotting time (ACT) ~300 seconds. Give 70-150 U/kg or 7000 U for women and 8000 U for men. If ACT not achieved give extra bolus of 2500-5000 U. Reduce heparin bolus to achieve ACT ~200 seconds if glycoprotein IIb/IIIa receptor agonist is to be used
- In high risk patients, abciximab as bolus and infusion should be given at least 10 minutes before angioplasty and stent placement and continued for 12 hours after procedure

### After procedure
- Start clopidogrel 300 mg orally, followed by 75 mg daily for 4 weeks
- Remove femoral sheath as soon as ACT falls below 150-180 seconds
- Heparin infusion is not routinely necessary after uncomplicated angioplasty

*Heparin infusion after a procedure is indicated if*
- Femoral sheath to be retained—Heparin infusion 1000-1200 U/hour until 4 hours before sheath is to be removed. Check ACT and remove sheath when ACT < 150 seconds
- Patients at high risk for in stent thrombosis
- Patients with other indications for anticoagulation, such as atrial fibrillation or mechanical heart valves

*Details given for unfractionated heparin, but low molecular weight heparin can be used as an alternative in percutaneous coronary interventions

## Further reading
- The Task Force on the management of acute coronary syndromes of the European Society of Cardiology. Management of acute coronary syndromes in patients presenting without persistent ST segment elevation. *Eur Heart J* 2002;23:1809-40
- Braunwald E, Antman EM, Beasley JW, Califf RM, Cheitlin MD, Hochman JS, et al. ACC/AHA 2002 guideline update for the management of patients with unstable angina and non-ST segment elevation myocardial infarction. *J Am Coll Cardiol* 2002;40:1366-74
- Fox KA, Poole-Wilson PA, Henderson RA, Clayton TC, Chamberlin DA, Shaw TR, et al for the Randomized Intervention Trial of Unstable Angina (RITA) Investigators. Interventional versus conservative treatment for patients with unstable angina or non-ST-elevation myocardial infarction: the British Heart Foundation RITA3 randomised trial. *Lancet* 2002;360:743-51
- Leon MB, Baim DS, Popma JJ, Gordon PC, Cutlip DE, Ho KK, et al for the Stent Anticoagulation Restenosis Study Investigators. A clinical trial comparing three antithrombotic-drug regimens after coronary-artery stenting. *N Engl J Med* 1998;339:1665-71
- Roffi M, Moliterno DJ, Meier B, Powers ER, Grines CL, DiBattiste PM, et al. Impact of different platelet glycoprotein IIb/IIIa receptor inhibitors among diabetic patients undergoing percutaneous coronary intervention: do tirofiban and Reopro give similar efficacy outcomes trial (TARGET) 1 year follow up? *Circulation* 2002;105:2730-6

The meta-analysis of trials comparing thrombolytic treatment with primary angioplasty is adapted from Weaver WD, et al, *JAMA* 1997;278:2093. The figure showing incidence of primary end point in patients treated with aspirin alone, aspirin and warfarin, or aspirin and ticlopidine after coronary artery stenting is adapted from Leon MB, et al, *N Engl J Med* 1998;339:1665-71. The figure showing the results from the PRISM-PLUS study is adapted from PRISM-PLUS Study Investigators. *N Engl J Med* 1998;338:1488-97. The figure showing the time course of cardiac biochemical markers is adapted from Wu AH, et al, *Clin Chem* 1999;45:1104-21. The figures of death or myocardial infarcton in patients with elevated troponins or negative troponin result, and the strategy for acute coronary syndromes are adapted from Bertrand ME, et al, *Eur Heart J* 2002;23:1809-40.

# 13 Antithrombotic therapy in chronic heart failure in sinus rhythm

Gregory Y H Lip, Bernard S P Chin

Chronic heart failure is one of the few remaining areas in cardiovascular medicine where the use of antithrombotic therapy remains controversial. This is largely because of conflicting outcomes from existing studies, a lack of appropriately conducted randomised clinical trials, and difficulty in defining the syndrome of heart failure and its thromboembolic complications.

## Stroke and systemic embolism in heart failure

Left ventricular dysfunction increases the risk of thrombosis and systemic embolism, and these thromboembolic events add to the high morbidity associated with this condition. In addition, ischaemic and thromboembolic events—particularly stroke, myocardial ischaemia, and myocardial infarction—contribute to the high hospital admission rates in these patients.

The incidence of thromboembolism and the factors associated with a high thromboembolic risk have been addressed in many studies, but the reported incidence of these events seems to vary between studies, depending on study methodology and populations. Retrospective analyses of recent heart failure trials have estimated this risk to be between 1.3% and 4.6% depending on the severity of heart failure. For example, mild to moderate chronic heart failure seems to be associated with an annual stroke risk of about 1.5% (V-HeFT and SOLVD studies), compared with an annual stroke risk in the general population of less than 0.5%. The annual risk of stroke increases to almost 5% in severe chronic heart failure. Evidence from the Framingham study shows that chronic heart failure is a major risk factor for stroke, second only to atrial fibrillation.

Long term oral anticoagulation is beneficial in certain groups of patients with chronic heart failure, but the role of anticoagulation for patients with chronic heart failure in general is less clear. For example, oral anticoagulation is extremely effective in reducing stroke risk and other embolic events in patients with atrial fibrillation and chronic heart failure. Indeed, there is a wide variation in the use of oral anticoagulants in patients with chronic heart failure.

Although oral anticoagulation reduces thromboembolic events in various cardiovascular diseases, the potential risks of bleeding must also be considered. Importantly, the control of

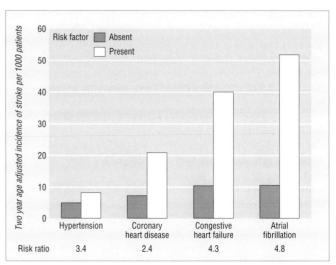

Two year age adjusted incidence of stroke for every thousand patients in the Framingham study

**The risk of recurrent strokes in heart failure patients is higher than with initial events. In heart failure patients, second and recurrent stroke rates may be as high as 9% every year**

---

**Rates of stroke, pulmonary embolism, myocardial infarction, and total mortality in recent heart failure trials**

| Study (NYHA) | NYHA | Mean ejection fraction | Mean age | Follow up (years) | Prevalence of atrial fibrillation (%) | Mean (SD) annual risk of events (%) | | | |
|---|---|---|---|---|---|---|---|---|---|
| | | | | | | Stroke | Pulmonary embolism | Myocardial infarction | Death |
| SOLVD | I-III | 0.25 | 60 | 3.3 | 6 | 3.8 (1.3) | 5.3 (1.6) | 9.6 (2.9) | 23.7 (7.2) |
| V-HeFT-I | II-III | 0.30 | 58 | 2.3 | 15 | 4.1 (1.8) | 5.6 (2.5) | – | 43.0 (18.7) |
| V-HeFT-II | II-III | 0.29 | 61 | 2.6 | 15 | 4.7 (1.8) | 5.7 (2.2) | 5.2 (2.0) | 34.7 (13.3) |
| CONSENSUS | III-IV | – | 71 | 0.5 | 50 | 2.3 (4.6) | – | – | 46.6 (44) |
| PROMISE | III-IV | 0.21 | 64 | 0.5 | – | 2.0 (3.5) | – | – | 27.1 (54) |
| SAVE | – | 0.30 | 59 | 3.5 | – | 4.6 (1.5) | – | 13.6 (3.9) | 18.9 (5.4) |

anticoagulation is reported to be more difficult, and bleeding complications commoner, in chronic heart failure because of hepatic congestion and potential drug interactions that may occur.

Studies have reported stroke incidences in heart failure of up to 11%. However, many of these trials were small, non-randomised and biased towards more severe disease. Importantly, atrial fibrillation was common among participants, many of whom did not receive warfarin during the period of follow up. Nevertheless, given that the risk of stroke in the general population aged 50-75 years is less than 0.5% a year, an estimated stroke incidence of 2% in patients with chronic heart failure represents a fourfold increased risk. With increasing age, the absolute risk of stroke rises, while its risk relative to the general population falls.

The commonest vascular occlusive event in heart failure is not stroke but myocardial infarction. Sudden cardiac death is common in heart failure and has been attributed to fatal arrhythmia. However, pathological studies of sudden cardiac deaths have detected fresh coronary thrombi in many cases, indicating that acute coronary occlusion may have been the primary event in the death. Many heart failure patients with myocardial infarction also die before reaching hospital. Hence, myocardial infarction and acute coronary occlusion may be more common in heart failure than estimated.

Sedentary patients with chronic heart failure patients are also at increased risk of developing venous thromboembolism, particularly in the legs. Pulmonary embolism can originate from deep vein thrombosis of the legs or, rarely, from a thrombus in the right ventricle.

### Left ventricular thrombus formation

Chronic heart failure patients in sinus rhythm are at high risk of ventricular thrombus formation because they fulfil Virchow's triad for thrombogenesis. These patients have:
- "Abnormal blood flow " with stasis, with low cardiac output, dilated cardiac chambers, and poor contractility of the heart;
- "Abnormal vessel walls", with endothelial damage or dysfunction or both;
- "Abnormal blood constituents", with abnormalities of haemostasis, platelets, and coagulation.

Autopsy and surgical studies have detected ventricular mural thrombi in 25-50% of heart failure patients. Such mural thrombi have been associated with increased mortality. In chronic heart failure with left ventricular dysfunction, abnormal wall motion leads to alterations in regional blood flow and inflow velocity, whereas impaired ventricular contractility results in further intracavitary blood stasis. Evidence exists for local platelet activation and cytokine recruitment, such as tumour necrosis factor, which can trigger the clotting cascade. This is particularly so after acute myocardial infarction, when high levels of catecholamines are circulating freely. Markers of endothelial injury and dysfunction are also elevated in heart failure, although in many cases these may be caused by underlying atherosclerosis. Endothelial damage promotes monocyte and platelet adhesion to the endothelium, predisposing to thrombosis in situ. The interplay of altered local flow characteristics, heightened clotting factors, and endothelial cell dysfunction gives rise to left ventricular thrombus formation.

Certain conditions are more likely to predispose to left ventricular thrombus formation. Patients with a dyskinetic left ventricular segment or left ventricular aneurysm and those who have had acute and extensive myocardial infarction involving the anterior wall are at highest risk. Left ventricular dilatation and severity of left ventricular dysfunction (measured by

### Stroke risk and heart failure

| | Annual risk |
|---|---|
| Stroke in general population aged 50-75 years | 0.5% |
| Stroke in mild chronic heart failure—NYHA II-III | 1.3-1.8% |
| Stroke in severe chronic heart failure—NYHA III-IV | 3.5-4.6% |
| Recurrent stroke rates in chronic heart failure | 9% |
| Stroke in atrial fibrillation | 4.5% |
| Stroke in atrial fibrillation and chronic heart failure | 8-12% |

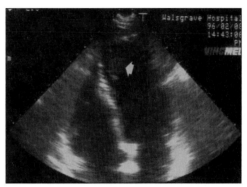

Apical thrombus in patient with poor left ventricular function

### Factors predisposing to prothrombotic state in heart failure

**Endothelial dysfunction**
- Impaired nitric oxide release
- Reduced anticoagulant status

**Altered flow characteristic**
- Left ventricular dilatation
- Abnormal left ventricular wall motion
- Left ventricular aneurysm
- Reduced pump action

**Altered coagulation**
- Increased platelet activation and aggregation
- Increased clotting
- Reduced fibrinolytic activity

**Neurohormonal and inflammatory activation**
- Increased catecholamines
- Increased inflammatory cytokines

ejection fraction) also correlate well with risk of thrombus formation. However, mitral regurgitation may have some protective effect.

### Risk factors for systemic embolisation

Given the high prevalence of left ventricular thrombus formation in patients with left ventricular aneurysm and heart failure, it is perhaps surprising that the rate of stroke in patients with documented left ventricular thrombi is low. This could be because of the difficulty in determining the presence of thrombus clinically. The best method is by cross sectional echocardiography, but this can only detect thrombi greater than 0.5 cm in diameter. Microthrombi that forms early in myocardial infarction and which pose a serious threat of embolism would not therefore be detected. Conversely, an organised chronic thrombus, which is more easily detectable on echocardiography is less likely to embolise.

A newly formed left ventricular thrombus is likely to embolise as are thrombi that are mobile, protruding, or pedunculated with a narrow stalk. Left ventricular thrombi present for more than three months would have undergone fibrous organisation and endothelialisation and so are more stable.

The only parameters shown by studies to achieve statistical significance as a predictor of thromboembolic events is peak oxygen uptake during symptom limited maximal exercise testing and the severity of heart failure (measured by left ventricular ejection fraction). The left ventricular ejection fraction is a powerful predictor of stroke in patients who have had a myocardial infarction. Patients with left ventricular ejection fraction less than 28% at particularly high risk. Furthermore, for every absolute decrease of 5% in left ventricular ejection fraction, the risk of stroke increases by 18%.

Patients with idiopathic dilated cardiomyopathy tend to have a higher rate of systemic thromboembolism than patients with ischaemic cardiomyocapthy. Only women with periparturm cardiomyopathy have higher risks of thromboembolism than patients with idiopathic dilated cardiomyopathy. Atrial fibrillation, age, and previous thromboembolic events are independent risk factors for stroke but confer further risks to patients with heart failure. Atrial fibrillation is associated with a stroke risk of about 5% every year.

## Antithrombotic treatment

### Warfarin

The need for oral anticoagulation in chronic heart failure has been inferred from mainly observational and retrospective studies of mortality from heart failure. In the PROMISE study, lower incidences of stroke were reported with anticoagulation (1.9% v 2.5%). In a follow up study of patients with idiopathic dilated cardiomyopathy, 18% of patients not taking warfarin had a stroke, whereas none occurred among the patients receiving warfarin over 11 years of follow up. Several studies of patients who had myocardial infarction showed that long term warfarin treatment to reduce rates of death, recurrent myocardial infarction, and stroke was effective.

Other studies have also shown that warfarin reduces mortality from sudden coronary death and recurrent myocardial infarction. Both the CONSENSUS and SOLVD studies showed that patients receiving warfarin had a lower mortality than those patients receiving antiplatelet treatment or those without antithrombotic therapy. In a retrospective survey of the SOLVD participants, anticoagulant monotherapy reduced the risk of sudden cardiac death by 32%. Among participants with non-ischaemic heart failure, this risk fell by

---

**Factors predisposing to left ventricular thrombus formation and embolisation**

**Left ventricular thrombus formation**
- After acute extensive myocardial infarction
- Acute anterior myocardial infarction
- Left ventricular aneurysm
- Left ventricular dilatation

**Systemic embolisation of left ventricular thrombi**
- New or acute thrombus (within two weeks of formation)
- Protruding segment
- Normal adjacent wall function

---

**Identifying risk factors that predispose to systemic embolisation of left ventricular thrombi is important because it allows patients at highest risk only to be treated. Currently, the identification of risk factors has been inferred from observational data of heart failure trials and smaller non-randomised studies**

---

**Major risk factors for cardioembolic stroke in chronic heart failure**

- Atrial fibrillation
- Mitral stenosis
- Prosthetic mechanical valves
- Presence of left ventricular mural thrombus
- Previous thromboembolism (stroke, pulmonary embolism, deep vein thrombosis)
- Poor left ventricular ejection fraction ($<28\%$)
- Acute left ventricular wall aneurysm
- Recent myocardial infarction
- Idiopathic dilated cardiomyopathy
- Infective endocarditis
- Atrial myxoma
- Reduced peak oxygen uptake at maximal exercise

**Studies comparing the effect of antithrombotic therapy in heart failure**

| Study | Treatment (anticoagulation *v* antiplatelet agents *v* placebo) | Stroke incidence every 100 patient years | Thromboembolic incidence every 100 patient years | Mortality |
|---|---|---|---|---|
| SOLVD | Aspirin *v* placebo | No effect | No effect | Lower with aspirin but benefit of enalapril blunted |
| SOLVD | Warfarin *v* placebo | No effect | No effect | Lower with warfarin |
| V-HeFT-I | Aspirin *v* warfarin *v* placebo | 0.5 *v* 1.9 *v* 2.0 | 0.5 *v* 2.9 *v* 2.7 | |
| CONSENSUS | Warfarin *v* placebo | ND | ND | Lower with warfarin |
| PROMISE | Warfarin *v* placebo | 1.9 *v* 2.9 | ND | |
| Fuster et al | Anticoagulants *v* placebo | ND | None *v* 3.5 | No effect |
| Katz et al | Aspirin *v* warfarin *v* placebo | 1.1 *v* 7.5 *v* 0.8 | ND | Lower with aspirin. No effect with warfarin |

ND = no data provided
Full references in Lip GYH, Gibbs CR *Quart J Med Cochrane Reviews* (see Further reading)

nearly 70%. The benefit of warfarin use is not uniform, as for example, the V-HeFT-1 Trial did not show any substantial benefit with warfarin use. Data from the SOLVD and V-HeFT studies were observational, without randomisation or control with respect to oral anticoagulation. In addition, interpretation of these data is potentially confounded—patients who were considered to be at highest risk of thromboembolism may have been treated with warfarin, and this would substantially reduce their long term risk of thromboembolic events.

Balanced against its potential benefits, warfarin increases the risk of intracranial haemorrhage by 0.3%. This complication increases with higher therapeutic targets (for example, INR 3.0-4.5). In heart failure patients with sinus rhythm, assuming a 2% risk of ischaemic stroke, warfarin use must reduce the risk by at least 20% to outweigh the threat of intracranial haemorrhages. Recurrent stroke rates in heart failure patients are also high (about 9% a year), and a reduction of only 10% would outweigh the risk of bleeding complications with warfarin. Secondary prevention of ischaemic strokes by warfarin in patients with heart failure should be considered.

Similarly, not all patients with documented left ventricular thrombi carry a high risk of embolisation. "High risk" patients such as those who have had an extensive acute anterior myocardial infarction or who show a new mural thrombus on cross sectional echocardiography should be considered for anticoagulation. Long term therapy (more than three months) is generally not recommended because of low embolisation rates from chronic left ventricular thrombi (unless the mass is mobile and pedunculated or other high risk factors exist).

Despite the limited evidence, some authorities recommend anticoagulation for patients with idiopathic dilated cardiomyopathy, whereas others using the postmyocardial infarction studies and data from SOLVD and CONSENSUS, advocate the use of warfarin in patients with ischaemic cardiomyopathy. A recent Cochrane systematic review does not recommend warfarin routinely for all heart failure patients in sinus rhythm because of conflicting conclusions from retrospective analyses and case series. More evidence is needed from randomised trials, such as the WATCH study (see later).

## Aspirin

Use of aspirin in heart failure is controversial, but it is commonly used in patients with chronic heart failure who are in sinus rhythm, because of its general efficacy as an antithrombotic agent in vascular disease. In addition, aspirin in general reduces the incidence of stroke and death in patients with recurrent episodes of cerebral ischaemia. Furthermore, aspirin has been shown to be moderately effective in reducing venous thrombosis and thromboembolism in patients undergoing hip surgery.

**Indications for warfarin treatment in chronic heart failure**

**Strongly recommended**
- Atrial fibrillation
- Previous ischaemic strokes
- New left ventricular mural thrombus formation
- Unstable, mobile left ventricular thrombus

**Individual consideration to be given**
- Idopathic dilated cardiomyopathies
- Poor left ventricular ejection fraction (<28%)
- Acute left ventricular aneurysm

**Not recommended**
- Sinus rhythm in absence of other risk factors
- Chronic left ventricular aneurysm
- Presence of chronic organised left ventricular mural thrombus

**Aspirin has been shown to reduce the incidence of myocardial infarction and death in men and women over 50 years, patients with unstable angina and myocardial infarction, and in patients with atherosclerotic cerebrovascular disease, whereas aspirin improves the patency rates of saphenous-vein aortocoronary bypass grafts**

Most trials of angiotensin converting enzyme (ACE) inhibitors, bar the SAVE study, have shown possible attenuation of their protective effects in heart failure after myocardial infarction when combined with aspirin. Several reasons have been put forward, not least because aspirin and ACE inhibitors exert effects on the same prostaglandin pathways. Concomitant aspirin can also limit sodium excretion and impair renal function in patients with chronic heart failure. The justification for using aspirin in chronic heart failure is strongest where an ischaemic aetiology is suspected. Indeed, aspirin reduces rates of death, recurrent myocardial infarction, and stroke when used in or shortly after acute myocardial infarction.

Although observational trials have shown a beneficial reduction of stroke with aspirin in patients with chronic heart failure, in general this reduction is less than that seen with warfarin. Two studies have shown aspirin to be more beneficial than warfarin in preventing strokes in heart failure. Both studies however were not randomised and it is possible that participants in the warfarin arm were more seriously ill or at higher risk of systemic embolism (for example, associated atrial fibrillation). Aspirin had no effect on mortality or risk of systemic embolism in patients with documented left ventriuclar thrombi.

A recent Cochrane systematic review concluded that there was conflicting evidence to support the use of antiplatelet drugs to reduce the incidence of thromboembolism in patients with chronic heart failure who are in sinus rhythm. There was also no direct evidence to indicate superior effects from oral anticoagulation, when compared with aspirin, in patients with chronic heart failure. Pending further evidence, aspirin cannot be recommended routinely for all patients with chronic heart failure (in sinus rhythm or atrial fibrillation) with or without left ventricular thrombi for the prevention of stroke and thromboembolism. Current guidelines should be tailored to individual risks and benefits.

Other antiplatelet drugs have not been represented in previous trials. Clopidogrel, which inhibits platelet function by inhibiting adenosine-induced platelet aggregation does not inhibit cyclo-oxygenase. Thus, it should not attenuate the beneficial actions of ACE inhibitors in the manner of aspirin. The large, ongoing randomised controlled WATCH study using clopidogrel, aspirin, and warfarin seeks to identify the optimal antithrombotic agent with the best risk:benefit ratio in the prevention of stroke and thromboembolism in heart failure.

# Acute heart failure

Patients with acute and decompensated heart failure not only have high levels of circulating catecholamines that may further activate the clotting cascade, but also tend to be less ambulatory and can be confined to bed or chair. The risk of venous thromboembolism is therefore increased and in fact, thromboembolic complications add to the burden of prolonged hospitalisation and mortality in these patients. Giving subcutaneous injections of unfractionated or low molecular weight heparin as prophylaxis can reduce the risk of venous thromboembolism, but trial evidence in chronic heart failure is lacking. No recent clinical trials show that warfarin or aspirin are effective in the primary prevention of venous thromboembolism or systemic complications in patients with acute heart failure who are in sinus rhythm.

## Further reading

- Al-Khadra AS, Salem DN, Rand WM, Udelson JE, Smith JJ, Konstam MA. Warfarin anticoagulation and survival: a cohort analysis from the Studies of Left Ventricular Dysfunction. *J Am Coll Cardiol* 1998; 31:749-53
- Cleland JG. Anticoagulant and antiplatelet therapy in heart failure. *Curr Opin Cardiol* 1997 12:276-87
- Dries DL, Rosenberg YD, Waclawiw MA, Domanski MJ. Ejection fraction and risk of thromboembolic events in patients with systolic dysfunction and sinus rhythm: evidence for gender differences in the studies of left ventricular dysfunction trials. *J Am Coll Cardiol* 1997; 29:1074-80
- Dunkman WB, Johnson GR, Carson PE, Bhat G, Farrell L, Cohn JN, for the V-HeFT VA Cooperative Studies Group. Incidence of thromboembolic events in congestive heart failure. *Circulation* 1993;87:VI194-101
- Lip GYH, Gibbs CR. Does heart failure confer a hypercoagulable state? Virchow's triad revisited. *J Am Coll Cardiol* 1999;5:1424-6
- Lip GYH, Gibbs CR. Anticoagulation for heart failure in sinus rhythm: a systematic Cochrane review. *Quart J Med* 2002;95:451-9
- Lip GYH, Gibbs CR. Antiplatelet agents versus control or anticoagulation for heart failure in sinus rhythm: a Cochrane systematic review. *Quart J Med* 2002;95:461-8
- Lip GYH. Intracardiac thrombus formation in cardiac impairment: the role of anticoagulant therapy. *Postgrad Med J* 1996;72:731-8
- Loh E, St. John Sutton M, Wun CC, et al. Ventricular dysfunction and the risk of stroke after myocardial infarction. *New Engl J Med* 1997;336:251-257
- Uretsky BF, Thygesen K, Armstrong PW, Cleland JG, Horowitz JD, Massie BM, et al. Acute coronary findings at autopsy in heart failure patients with sudden death: results from the assessment of treatment with lisinopril and survival (ATLAS) trial. *Circulation* 2000;102:611-6

We thank Professor JG Cleland (University of Hull, United Kingdom), for helpful comments during the preparation of this review

The figure showing the two year adjusted incidence of stroke in the Framingham study is adapted from Wolfe CD et al. *Stroke* 1991;22:983

# 14 Antithrombotic therapy in special circumstances. I–pregnancy and cancer

Bernd Jilma, Sridhar Kamath, Gregory Y H Lip

## Antithrombotic therapy during pregnancy

Pregnancy predisposes to venous thromboembolism for several reasons. These include a change in the balance between procoagulant and anticoagulant factors in the blood. Any conditions that predispose a woman to thromboembolism when she is not pregnant will also predispose her to thromboembolism when she is pregnant.

Generally, antithrombotic therapy started in a non-pregnant patient for a particular disorder needs to be continued during the pregnancy and in the puerperium. The use and type of antithrombotic therapy depends on the risk:benefit ratio, taking into consideration the potential harm to the mother and the fetus.

The potential risks of antithrombotic therapy during pregnancy can be divided into maternal and fetal risks, and include teratogenicity and bleeding. Unfractionated heparin and low molecular weight heparins do not cross the placenta and are probably safe for the fetus, although bleeding at the uteroplacental junction is possible. Nevertheless, data are sparse for low molecular weight heparin, with no reliable comparative trials or convincing dose assessment.

In contrast to heparin, coumarin derivatives cross the placenta and can cause both bleeding in the fetus and teratogenicity. Coumarin derivatives can cause an embryopathy (which consists of nasal hypoplasia or stippled epiphyses or both) after in utero exposure during the first trimester of pregnancy. In addition, central nervous system abnormalities can occur after exposure to such drugs during any trimester. The main risk of embryopathy occurs if coumarin derivatives are taken between six weeks and 12 weeks of gestation. At the time of delivery, the anticoagulant effect in the fetus can lead to bleeding in the neonate.

Heparin and low molecular weight heparins are not secreted into breast milk and can probably be given safely to nursing mothers. High dose aspirin should be avoided, as it could (theoretically) impair platelet function and produce hypoprothrombinaemia in the infant, if neonatal vitamin K stores are low, as well as cause Reye's syndrome. Warfarin does not induce an anticoagulant effect in an infant who is breast fed and therefore could be used safely in the postpartum period; thus, patients who are receiving long term heparin treatment could be switched over to warfarin post partum if and when considered appropriate. With regard to other agents, phenindione should be avoided, and acenocoumarol requires prophylactic vitamin K for the infant.

### Venous thrombosis and pulmonary embolism

Antithrombotic prophylaxis for the prevention of venous thromboembolic disorders in pregnancy is indicated when a patient has experienced a previous thromboembolic episode or is considered to be at particularly high risk because of a predisposing condition.

Unfractionated heparin 5000 IU twice daily is generally adequate in non-pregnant women. Heparin requirements can be highly variable in pregnancy. A once daily dose of low

---

**Disorders during pregnancy for which antithrombotic therapy is commonly considered**

- Prophylaxis and treatment of venous thromboembolism
- Prophylaxis in patients with valvar disease (for example, mitral stenosis)
- Prophylaxis in patients with mechanical prosthetic valves
- Antiphospholipid syndrome
- Prophylaxis against pregnancy induced hypertension and intrauterine growth retardation

---

**Potential risks of antithrombotic therapy during pregnancy**

**Maternal disadvantages and risks**

*Unfractionated heparin*
- Haemorrhage (uteroplacental, especially during labour)
- Heparin induced thrombocytopenia
- Osteoporosis
- Regular monitoring

*Low molecular weight heparin*
- Bleeding risk, especially during labour

*Warfarin*
- Bleeding
- Regular monitoring

**Risk to the fetus or child**

*Heparin*
- Seems to be safe

*Low molecular weight heparin*
- Seems to be safe

*Warfarin*
- Embryopathy, especially if mother is exposed between 6 and 12 weeks
- Central nervous system malformations during any time of the gestation

*Low dose aspirin*
- Potential risk of birth defects and bleeding risk in the first trimester
- Safe in second and third trimester

---

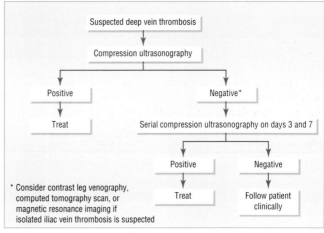

Diagnosis of suspected deep vein thrombosis in pregnancy

molecular weight heparin is a useful alternative to unfractionated heparin and has been shown to be safe and effective in pregnancy.

Patients who develop thromboembolism during pregnancy could be treated initially with at least five days of intravenous heparin treatment, followed by a twice daily subcutaneous dose of unfractionated heparin. The dose is adjusted by maintaining the activated partial thromboplastin time (APTT) within the therapeutic levels. Heparin could temporarily be stopped immediately before delivery and then resumed in the postpartum period to minimise the risk of haemorrhage during labour. The duration of antithrombotic therapy in the postpartum period should be maintained for a minimum of three months, possibly up to six months.

### Patients with prosthetic heart valves
The precise safety of warfarin during pregnancy continues to be debated, but it is probably appropriate to withhold warfarin between six and 12 weeks of gestation and for the latter half of the third trimester, because of the risk of causing embryopathy and postpartum haemorrhage respectively. Based on this, the recommended options for use of antithrombotic therapy in patients with a mechanical heart valve during pregnancy include:
- Adjusted dose of unfractionated heparin twice daily to maintain the APTT within therapeutic range, or low molecular weight heparin throughout the pregnancy
- Warfarin throughout the pregnancy, except for the first trimester (either for the entire trimester or between six and 12 weeks) and for the latter half of the third trimester (when warfarin should be replaced by unfractionated or low molecular weight heparin).

The risks and benefits of this approach should be explained to patients, who should be allowed to make an informed choice. There are real concerns over the incidence of abortions and fetal malformations in patients treated with warfarin in the first trimester. Concerns over long term heparin treatment in pregnant women include heparin induced thrombocytopenia and osteoporosis.

Prepregnancy counselling is vital for patients who are receiving long term warfarin treatment, and a cardiologist and obstetrician should explain the risks to patients. Patients who are established on long term warfarin treatment and plan to become pregnant could then take twice daily heparin before getting pregnant. Alternatively, and assuming that the risk of warfarin to the fetus in the first six weeks of gestation is not worrisome, they could continue taking warfarin and have frequent checks to see if they are pregnant. If they are, they should immediately switch over to heparin. Again, close liaison between obstetrician, midwife, general practitioner, cardiologist, and neonatologist is vital.

### Antiphospholipid syndrome
Antiphospholipid syndrome predisposes a pregnant woman to thromboembolism and pregnancy losses. Abortion in a previous pregnancy predisposes to further abortions or stillbirths in subsequent pregnancies. A combination of aspirin and heparin to prolong the APTT to within the therapeutic range (APTT ratio 2.0-3.0) throughout the pregnancy would substantially decrease pregnancy losses and other complications. However, one recent trial suggested that low dose aspirin (75 mg) may suffice (see box), but small numbers merit some caution pending further data.

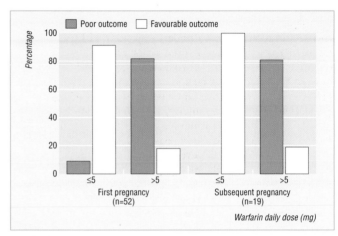

Distribution of warfarin dose and poor outcome according to order of pregnancy. The risk of pregnancy complication in patients treated with warfarin is higher when the mean daily dose exceeds 5 mg (P<0.001)

**Antiphospholipid syndrome in pregnancy: a randomised controlled trial of aspirin _v_ aspirin plus heparin**

|  | Low dose aspirin (n=47) | Low dose aspirin plus heparin (n=51) |
|---|---|---|
| Live birth rate (%) | 72 | 78 |
| Mean (SD) birth weight (g): | 3221 (781) | 3127 (657) |
|   Range | 890-5300 | 718-4319 |
| Gestation at delivery (%): |  |  |
|   <30 weeks | 1 | 1 |
|   30-36 weeks | 3 | 1 |
|   >36 weeks | 30 | 38 |
| Embryo loss (%) | 9 | 3 |
| Fetal loss (%) | 4 | 8 |

**Antithrombotic therapy in antiphospholipid syndrome**

| Scenario | Management |
|---|---|
| History of pregnancy loss | Aspirin plus heparin (APTT in therapeutic range) |
| History of thromboembolism but no pregnancy loss | Heparin alone (APTT in therapeutic range) |
| No history of adverse events | Heparin alone 5000 IU twice daily; close observation |

## Pre-eclampsia and intrauterine growth retardation

On the basis of small, retrospective studies, low dose aspirin (< 150 mg daily) was thought to be useful as prophylaxis in patients with a history of pre-eclampsia and intrauterine growth retardation in preventing similar adverse events during the current pregnancy. However, a large (nearly 10 000 women) randomised controlled trial (CLASP) of aspirin 60 mg compared with placebo, reported that, although aspirin was associated with a 12% reduction in the incidence of pre-eclampsia, this was not significant nor was there any substantial impact on intrauterine growth retardation, stillbirth, or neonatal death. Thus, routine use of low dose aspirin is not recommended. However, some experts recommend its use in patients who are liable to develop early onset (before 32 weeks) pre-eclampsia or in high risk groups for pre-eclampsia, such as women with type 1 diabetes, chronic hypertension, multiple pregnancies, or previous pre-eclampsia. However, the safety of higher doses of aspirin and aspirin ingestion during the first trimester remains uncertain.

# Antithrombotic therapy in cancer

Venous thromboembolism is a frequent complication in patients with cancer, and it is a common clinical problem. It can even precede the diagnosis of cancer by months or years. Patients with cancer are nearly twice as likely to die from pulmonary embolism in hospital as those with benign disease, and about 60% of these deaths occur prematurely. Thromboembolism seems to be particularly predominant in patients with mucinous carcinoma of the pancreas, lung, or gastrointestinal tract. This may be because cancer can be associated with raised levels of procoagulants such as fibrinogen, von Willebrand factor, and tissue factor, as well as excess platelet activity. Raised levels of plasminogen activator inhibitor are often present, and this will impair fibrinolysis. Therapeutic interventions in patients with cancer, such as surgery, standard chemotherapy, or hormone based treatment (such as oestrogens for prostatic cancer), further increase the risk for thrombosis. One reason for this may be that certain types of chemotherapy impair the natural anticoagulant properties of the endothelium, thus promoting a procoagulant state. Unfortunately, no standardised protocols exist for the management of patients with cancer and the approaches vary.

## Primary prophylaxis

In patients with cancer who are confined to bed or having low risk surgical procedures a low dose of unfractionated heparin or low molecular weight heparin is administered subcutaneously, along with physical measures, as primary prophylaxis to reduce thromboembolic risk. Patients having major abdominal or pelvic surgery for cancer are recommended to receive adjusted dose heparin, low molecular weight heparin, or oral anticoagulants (therapeutic international normalised ratio (INR) 2.0-3.0) similar to those for major orthopaedic surgery.

A low dose warfarin regimen is recommended for patients receiving chemotherapy or those with indwelling venous catheters to decrease the incidence of thromboembolism. For example, one double blind randomised study of patients with metastatic breast cancer receiving chemotherapy showed that a very low dose (1 mg/day) of warfarin for six weeks followed by a dose to maintain the INR at 1.3-1.9 was effective. Low dose low molecular weight heparin (for example, daltaparin 2500 IU/day) is an alternative for patients with indwelling venous catheters.

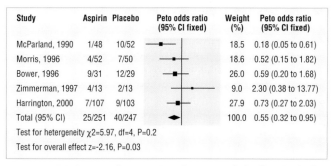

| Study | Aspirin | Placebo | Peto odds ratio (95% CI fixed) | Weight (%) | Peto odds ratio (95% CI fixed) |
|---|---|---|---|---|---|
| McParland, 1990 | 1/48 | 10/52 | | 18.5 | 0.18 (0.05 to 0.61) |
| Morris, 1996 | 4/52 | 7/50 | | 18.6 | 0.52 (0.15 to 1.82) |
| Bower, 1996 | 9/31 | 12/29 | | 26.0 | 0.59 (0.20 to 1.68) |
| Zimmerman, 1997 | 4/13 | 2/13 | | 9.0 | 2.30 (0.38 to 13.77) |
| Harrington, 2000 | 7/107 | 9/103 | | 27.9 | 0.73 (0.27 to 2.03) |
| Total (95% CI) | 25/251 | 40/247 | | 100.0 | 0.55 (0.32 to 0.95) |
| Test for hetergeneity χ2=5.97, df=4, P=0.2 | | | | | |
| Test for overall effect z=-2.16, P=0.03 | | | | | |

Effect of aspirin in preventing pre-eclampsia: meta-analysis of randomised trials showing numbers of cases of pre-eclampsia

---

## Virchow's triad* in cancer

**Abnormal blood flow**
- Increased viscosity and turbulence
- Increased stasis from immobility

**Abnormal blood constituents**
- Increased platelet activation and aggregation
- Increased procoagulant factors
- Decreased anticoagulant and fibrinolytic factors

**Abnormal blood vessel wall**
- Damaged or dysfunctional endothelium
- Loss of anticoagulant nature
- Possibly angiogenesis

*For thrombogenesis (thrombus formation) there needs to be a triad of abnormalities (abnormal blood flow, abnormal blood constituents, and abnormal blood vessel wall)

---

## Risk factors for thromboembolism in patients with cancer

- Prolonged immobility
- Chemotherapy
- Surgical procedures
- Indwelling vascular catheters

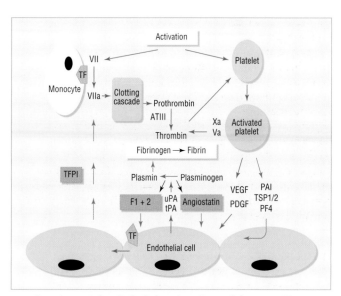

Overview of coagulation, fibrinolysis, and angiogenesis in cancer. The activation of platelets leads to their swelling and the release of angiogenic factors. These affect the vascular endothelia of healing and tumour tissues. The blue arrows facilitate angiogenesis and the red arrows are inhibitory (ATIII=antithrombin III, F1 + 2=prothrombin fragments, PAI=plasminogen activator inhibitor, PDGF=platelet derived growth factor, PF4=platelet factor 4, TF=tissue factor, TFPI=tissue factor pathway inhibitor, TSP1/2=thrombospondin 1 and 2, tPA=tissue type plasminogen activator, uPA=urokinase type plasminogen activator, VEGF=vascular endothelial growth factor)

## Treatment and secondary prevention

Patients with cancer who develop a thromboembolism should be treated in a similar manner to patients without cancer. An initial period of therapeutic unfractionated heparin or low molecular weight heparin which is overlapped and followed by warfarin for a minimum of three months is recommended. Anticoagulation should be continued in patients who have active disease or who receive chemotherapy while these risk factors last. The dose should maintain an INR of between 2.0 and 3.0.

## Risk of haemorrhage

Patients with cancer who are receiving antithrombotic therapy are thought to be at higher risk of bleeding than patients without cancer. This assumption has been disputed, however, in light of the evidence from some studies in which the risk of major bleeding did not differ greatly between the two groups of patients. For practical purposes, the recommended therapeutic levels of anticoagulation remain the same (for example, if warfarin, then INR 2.0-3.0) as long as patients are educated about the risks and the anticoagulation levels are strictly monitored. The propensity for chemotherapy to be given in cycles or boluses, followed by periods free of chemotherapy, seems likely to frustrate attempts to maintain the INR within its target range.

Definite conclusions cannot be drawn about the safety of antithrombotic therapy in patients with primary or secondary brain malignancy. Some small studies report that it is probably safe to give these patients anticoagulants. However, definite decisions about anticoagulation in such patients have to be individualised and carefully considered. Anticoagulation should probably be avoided in patients with brain metastasis because of the chances of renal cell carcinoma or melanoma, as these tumours are highly vascular.

## Recurrent venous thromboembolism

Patients with cancer are at a higher risk than non-cancer patients of recurrence of thromboembolism despite adequate anticoagulation. Again, no strict evidence based guidelines exist for the management of these patients. The recommended options include maintenance of a higher level of anticoagulation (INR 3.0 to 4.5), substitution with adjusted dose heparin or low molecular weight heparin (some evidence suggests heparin is probably better in this situation), and placement of inferior venacaval filters with or without anticoagulation.

The figure showing diagnosis of deep vein thrombosis is adapted from Chan W-S et al, *Thromb Res* 2002;107:85-91. The table showing the results of aspirin *v* aspirin plus heparin in treating antiphospholipid syndrome in pregnancy is adapted from Farquharson RG et al, *Obstet Gynecol* 2002;100:408-13. The table showing Virchow's triad in cancer is adapted from Lip GYH et al, *Lancet Oncol* 2002;3:27-34. The histogram showing distribution of warfarin dose and poor outcome according to order of pregnancy is adapted from Cotrufo M et al, *Obstet Gynecol* 2002;99:35-40. The meta-analysis showing the effect of aspirin in preventing pre-eclampsia is adapted from Coomarasamy A et al, *Obstet Gynecol* 2001;98:861-6. The figure showing the overview of coagulation, fibrinolysis, and angiogenesis in cancer is adapted from Nash G et al, *Lancet Oncol* 2001;2:608-13.

## Concerns about antithrombotic therapy in cancer

- Recurrent venous thromboembolism
- Increased tendency for minor and major bleeds
- Inconsistency in therapeutic anticoagulant levels
- Procoagulant effects of chemotherapy (for example, endothelial cell dysfuntion)

## Further reading

- Barbour LA. Current concepts of anticoagulation therapy in pregnancy. *Obstet Gynecol Clin North Am* 1997;24:499-521
- CLASP (Collaborative Low-dose Aspirin Study in Pregnancy) Collaborative Group. CLASP: a randomised trial of low-dose aspirin for the prevention and treatment of pre-eclampsia among 9364 pregnant women. *Lancet* 1994;343:619-29
- Cumming AM, Shiach CR. The investigation and management of inherited thrombophilia. *Clin Lab Haem* 1999;21:77-92
- Coomarasamy A, Papaioannou S, Gee H, Khan KS. Aspirin for the prevention of preeclampsia in women with abnormal uterine artery Doppler: a meta-analysis. *Obstet Gynecol* 2001;98:861-6
- Cotrufo M, De Feo M, De Santo LS, Romano G, Della Corte A, Renzilli A, et al. Risk of warfarin during pregnancy with mechanical valve prostheses. *Obstet Gynecol* 2002;99:35-40
- Ginsberg JS, Greer I, Hirsh J. Use of antithrombotic agents during pregnancy. *Chest* 2001:119;S122-31
- Farquharson RG, Quenby S, Greaves M. Antiphospholipid syndrome in pregnancy: a randomized, controlled trial of treatment. *Obstet Gynecol* 2002;100:408-13
- Letai A, Kuter DJ. Cancer, coagulation, and anticoagulation. *Oncologist* 1999;4:443-9
- Levine M, Hirsh J, Gent M, Arnold A, Warr D, Falanga A, et al. Double-blind randomised trial of a very-low-dose warfarin for prevention of thromboembolism in stage IV breast cancer. *Lancet* 1994;343:886-9
- Lip GYH, Chin BSP, Blann AD. Cancer and the prothrombotic state. *Lancet Oncol* 2002;3:27-34
- Prandoni P. Antithrombotic strategies in patients with cancer. *Thromb Haemost* 1997;78:141-4
- Sanson BJ, Lensing AW, Prins MH, Ginsberg JS, Barkagan ZS, Lavanne-Pardlonge E, et al. Safety of low-molecular-weight heparin in pregnancy: a systematic review. *Thromb Haemost* 1999;81:668-72
- Chan W-S, Ginsberg JS. Diagnosis of deep vein thrombosis and pulmonary embolism in pregnancy. *Thromb Res* 2002;107:85-91

# 15  Antithrombotic therapy in special circumstances. II–children, thrombophilia, and miscellaneous conditions

Bernd Jilma, Sridhar Kamath, Gregory Y H Lip

## Treatments for children

Most of the recommendations on antithrombotic therapy in children are based on the extrapolation of results from randomised studies of adults or from small cross sectional, and mainly retrospective, clinical studies of children. Although antithrombotic therapy in children usually follows the same indications as in adults, the distribution of diseases requiring antithrombotic therapy differs in the paediatric population. For example, some predisposing factors for thromboembolism are encountered only in paediatric populations. Most of the indications for antithrombotic therapy in children arise because of an underlying medical disorder or an intervention for the management of the disorder. Management of antithrombotic therapy in children differs from that in adults because of ongoing changes in physiology that may alter the thrombotic process and potentially influence the response of the body to antithrombotic therapy.

### Drug treatments

#### Antiplatelet treatment
Aspirin, dipyramidole, and indomethacin are probably the most used antiplatelet treatments among children. Low doses of aspirin (antiplatelet doses) usually have minimal side effects in children, but in general aspirin should not be prescribed to children aged < 16 years unless there are compelling clinical indications. The particular concerns about Reye's syndrome usually seem to be related to higher doses of aspirin (> 40 mg/kg).

#### Heparin
Heparin is probably the most commonly used antithrombotic drug in children. Varying concentrations of antithrombin in the body during different developmental stages mean that the therapeutic concentration of heparin in children has to be maintained by regular checks of the activated partial thromboplastin time (APTT) or anti-Xa concentrations. The recommended therapeutic level of APTT is the one which corresponds to a heparin concentration of 0.2-0.4 U/ml or an anti-Xa concentration of 0.3-0.7 U/ml.

In children, the advantages of low molecular weight heparin over unfractionated heparin are similar to those in adults. In addition, low molecular weight heparin may be preferred for children with difficult venous access because regular blood checks to monitor the therapeutic levels are not mandatory. The recommended therapeutic dose of a low molecular weight heparin is the one that reflects the plasma anti-Xa concentrations of 0.5-1.0 U/ml four to six hours after injection.

#### Oral anticoagulants
Certain problems are associated with the use of oral anticoagulants in children. Sensitivity to oral anticoagulants changes during different phases of life, especially during infancy, because of varying concentrations of vitamin K and vitamin K dependent proteins in the body. Neonates (during the first month

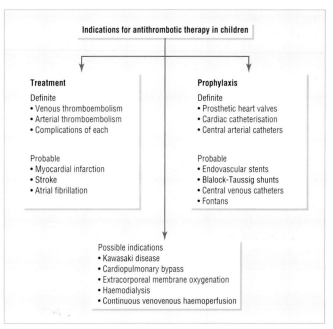

Indications for antithrombotic therapy in children

**Adjusting low molecular weight heparin in children**

| Anti-Xa level (U/ml) | Hold next dose? | Dose change? | Repeat anti-Xa measurement |
|---|---|---|---|
| <0.35 | No | Increase by 25% | 4 hours after next dose |
| 0.35-0.49 | No | Increase by 10% | 4 hours after next dose |
| 0.5-1.0 | No | No | Next day, then 1 week later, and monthly thereafter while receiving reviparin-Na treatment (4 hours after morning dose) |
| 1.1-1.5 | No | Decrease by 20% | Before next dose |
| 1.6-2.0 | 3 hours | Decrease by 30% | Before next dose then 4 hours after next dose |
| >2.0 | Until anti-Xa 0.5 U/ml | Decrease by 40% | Before next dose, then every 12 hours until anti-Xa level <0.5 U/ml |

of life) are especially sensitive because of their relative deficiency of vitamin K, and therefore warfarin should be avoided in such patients if possible. However, formula fed infants are resistant to oral anticoagulants because of a high concentration of vitamin K in their diet. In general, young children need more oral anticoagulation for each kilogram of body weight than older children and adults. Poor venous access (for international normalised ratio (INR) checks) and non-compliance are added problems of anticoagulation in children.

Recommended therapeutic ranges and duration of anticoagulation for a variety of disorders in children are usually similar to those for adults.

*Thrombolytic treatment*
Thrombolytic treatment is used primarily for maintaining catheter patency and in the management of thromboembolism that threatens the viability of the affected organ. Thrombolytic drugs are used locally or systemically and their concentration can be monitored with plasma fibrinogen levels or total clotting time. Decreased plasma plasminogen levels in newborns may reduce the thrombolytic actions of the drugs. Thrombolytic drugs pose similar risks to children as to adults.

**Venous thromboembolism**
Venous thromboembolism in children usually occurs secondary to an underlying disorder, such as in the upper arm secondary to a central venous line being inserted. Such lines are usually placed for intensive care management and treatment of cancer. The patency of these lines is traditionally maintained through therapeutic local instillation of urokinase for blocked lines or prophylactic intermittent boluses of heparin (which have doubtful efficacy).

Established venous thromboembolism requires removal of the predisposing factor and anticoagulation similar to that in adults (standard heparin for five days followed by maintenance with oral anticoagulation for at least three months). Oral anticoagulation can be started on the same day as heparin. Low molecular weight heparin is a useful option for maintaining anti-Xa level of 0.5-1.0 U/ml. Patients with a first recurrence of venous thromboembolism or with an initial episode with continuing risk factors either could be closely monitored for any early signs of thromboembolism or should be given anticoagulant drugs prophylactically after the period of initial therapeutic anticoagulation for the episode. Patients with a second recurrence of venous thromboembolism or with a first recurrence with continuing risk factors should be given anticoagulants for life, as in adults.

**Arterial thromboembolism**
The usual predisposing factors include placement of central and peripheral arterial catheters for cardiac catheterisation and intensive care settings. A bolus of heparin (50-150 U/kg) at the time of arterial puncture and continuous low dose heparin infusion are common methods for cardiac and umbilical artery catheterisation, respectively.

**Prosthetic heart valves**
Oral anticoagulation is needed in children with mechanical heart valves. An INR of 2.5-3.5 is recommended as the target range. Patients who are predisposed to high risk of thromboembolism despite anticoagulation treatment and those with thromboembolism while taking warfarin could benefit from the addition of antiplatelet drugs, such as aspirin (6-20 mg/kg/day) or dipyridamole (2-5 mg/kg/day), to oral anticoagulation.

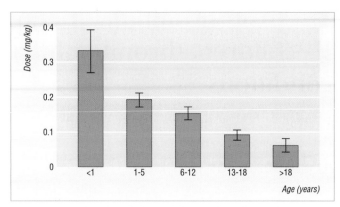

Effect of age on dose of warfarin needed to sustain an international normalised ratio (INR) of 2.0-3.0 in 262 children. Younger children required significantly more warfarin than older children (P<0.001)

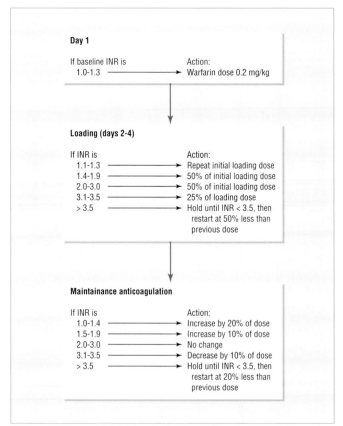

Protocol for oral anticoagulation treatment to maintain an INR ratio of 2.0-3.0 for children

**Commonly used drugs in children that affect INR values**

| Drug | Usual effect on INR |
| --- | --- |
| Amiodarone | Increase |
| Aspirin | Increase or no change |
| Amoxicillin | Slight increase |
| Cefaclor | Increase |
| Carbamazepine | Decrease |
| Phenytoin | Decrease |
| Phenobarbital | Decrease |
| Cloxacillin | Increase |
| Prednisone | Increase |
| Co-trimoxazole | Increase |
| Ranitidine | Increase |

## Other cardiac disorders

No universally accepted guidelines or randomised trials exist for the antithrombotic therapy in patients undergoing operations where there is risk of thromboembolism (such as Blalock-Taussig shunts, Fontan operations, and endovascular stents). A variety of antithrombotic regimens have been used after these operations, including intraoperative heparin only and intraoperative heparin followed by oral anticoagulation or aspirin.

## Hereditary prothrombotic states

Deficiencies of protein C, protein S, or antithrombin III and factor V Leiden mutation can lead to thromboembolism especially in the presence of a secondary risk factor. Homozygous deficiency of these proteins could lead to fatal purpura fulminans in newborns, which is treated immediately by rapid replacement of these factors with fresh frozen plasma or protein concentrates. This is followed by careful initiation of lifelong oral anticoagulation to maintain the INR at higher levels of 3.0-4.5. Heterozygous patients could be given prophylactic antithrombotic therapy during exposure to secondary risk factors or be followed up with close observation.

# Antithrombotic therapy in thrombophilia and miscellaneous conditions

A detailed discussion of management of thrombophilic disorders is beyond the scope of this article. The guidelines on the management of these disorders are based on small and non-controlled series of patients because of the paucity of randomised trials (as reviewed by the Haemostasis and Thrombosis Task Force in 2001).

Inherited thrombophilic disorders are genetically determined, and most of the affected patients are heterozygotes. Homozygotes are extremely rare. Antithrombin III, protein C, and protein S are produced in the liver and act by inactivating coagulation factors. Deficiency of these proteins could lead to uncontrolled activation of the coagulation cascade and therefore thromboembolism.

Activated protein C resistance is the commonest inherited thrombophilic disorder and accounts for 20-50% of cases. Antithrombin III deficiency is the rarest of the mentioned inherited thrombophilic disorders but carries the highest thrombogenic risk. High plasma concentration of homocysteine is linked to genetic enzyme deficiencies and low plasma concentrations of folate and vitamin B-6, and an investigation of vitamin B-12 metabolism is warranted.

Though thrombophilic disorders predispose patients to thromboembolism, the routine use of anticoagulation for primary prophylaxis entails greater risks than benefit (except probably in homozygotes). Therefore primary prophylaxis is warranted only in the presence of a second risk factor, and for as long as the risk factor lasts. Common predisposing factors that require prophylaxis include surgery, immobilisation, pregnancy and the puerperium, and oral contraception.

Special caution is needed when giving anticoagulation to patients with protein C deficiency. Because protein C is a vitamin K dependent factor, the administration of warfarin could lead to sudden decrease in protein C before any noticeable decrease in coagulation factors. This could cause enhanced thrombosis and diffuse skin necrosis. This adverse response can be avoided by gradual initiation of oral anticoagulation with low doses of warfarin, preferably overlapped by adequate heparinisation. In cases of severe deficiency, replacement of protein C is indicated before starting warfarin.

## Common thrombophilic disorders

**Inherited**
- Antithrombin III deficiency
- Protein C deficiency
- Protein S deficiency
- Activated protein C resistance (factor V Leiden mutation)
- Inherited hyperhomocysteinaemia
- Raised factor VIII levels
- Prothrombin gene G20210 A variant

**Acquired**
- Antiphospholipid syndrome
- Acquired hyperhomocysteinaemia

## Guidelines for antithrombotic therapy in inherited thrombophilia*

| Indication | Treatment |
|---|---|
| *Primary prophylaxis* | |
| Any surgery | Unfractionated heparin subcutaneously 5000 IU three times daily |
| Malignancy or orthopaedic surgery | Unfractionated heparin subcutaneously 5000 IU three times daily, possibly with replacement of deficient factors |
| Pregnancy | Unfractionated heparin subcutaneously 5000 IU three times daily |
| Pregnancy in antithrombin III deficiency | Therapeutic dose of unfractionated heparin to prolong APTT or dose adjusted warfarin (INR 2.0-3.0), except during first trimester and latter part of third trimester, when unfractionated heparin is used |
| Puerperium (for 4-6 weeks) | Unfractionated heparin subcutaneously 5000 IU three times daily or dose adjusted warfarin (INR 2.0-3.0) |
| *Secondary prophylaxis* | |
| First episode of thrombosis | Dose adjusted warfarin for 6 months |
| First episode of life threatening thrombosis, multiple deficiencies, continuing predisposing factor | Lifelong oral anticoagulation |
| Recurrent thrombosis | Lifelong oral anticoagulation |
| *Treatment of established thrombosis* | |
| Treatment of acute thrombosis | Unfractionated heparin to prolong APTT followed by oral anticoagulation treatment, possibly with replacement of the deficient factors |

*For full guidelines see Haemostasis and Thrombosis Task Force, *Br J Haematol* 2001;114:512-28
Low molecular weight heparins are increasingly used as alternatives to unfractionated heparin

Little evidence exists to support the use of antithrombotic agents in hyperhomocysteinaemia. Although replacement of folic acid and vitamin B-6 has been shown to reduce plasma homocysteine levels, no study has found reduction in thromboembolic events with this intervention.

### Antiphospholipid syndrome
The long term prognosis for this syndrome is influenced by the risk of recurrent thrombosis. As with other thrombophilic disorders, primary prophylaxis is not indicated in the absence of other risk factors. A patient with one episode of thrombosis is at considerable risk of further thrombosis and should be given lifelong anticoagulation with warfarin as secondary prophylaxis. The target INR should be 2.0-3.0 (although some authorities advocate a higher INR level ($\geqslant$3.0)). Patients with this syndrome may be relatively resistant to warfarin and so will need high doses. However, some authorities believe that the antiphospholipid antibodies interfere with the generation of the INR and lead to spurious results. Consequently, other routes to monitoring anticoagulation may be needed.

Low molecular weight heparin is used increasingly in patients with various thrombophilia and seems to be safe and reliable.

### Kawasaki disease
Aspirin continues to be used in Kawasaki disease despite a lack of unequivocal evidence from randomised trials of its benefit in reducing coronary artery aneurysm or thrombosis. Aspirin is used in anti-inflammatory doses (50-100 mg/kg/day) during the acute stage of the disease, followed by antiplatelet doses (1-5 mg/kg/day) for seven weeks or longer.

The figure showing effect of age on dose of warfarin in 262 children is adapted from Streif W et al, *Curr Opin Pediatr* 1999;11:56-64. The diagram of protocol for oral anticoagulation for children and the tables showing adjustment of low molecular weight heparin in children and commonly used drugs in children are adapted from Monagle P et al, *Chest* 2001;119:S344-70. The guidelines for antithrombotic therapy in inherited thrombophilia are adapted from the Haemostasis and Thrombosis Task Force, *Br J Haemotol* 2001;114:512-28. The box of recommendations from the College of Amercian Pathologists consensus conference on diagnostic issues in thrombophilia is adapted from Olson JD, *Arch Pathol Lab Med* 2002;126:1277-80.

### Recommendations from the College of American Pathologists consensus conference XXXVI: diagnostic issues in thrombophilia
- Patients, and especially asymptomatic family members, should provide informed consent before thrombophilia testing is performed
- Individuals testing positive for a thrombophilia need counselling on:
  *Risks of thrombosis* to themselves and their family members
  *Importance of early recognition* of the signs and symptoms of venous thromboembolism that would require immediate medical attention
  *Risks and benefits* of antithrombotic prophylaxis in situations in which their risk of thrombosis is increased, such as surgery or pregnancy
- Laboratory testing for other inherited and acquired thrombophilias should be considered even after the identification of a known thrombophilia because more than one thrombophilia could coexist, compounding the risk for thrombosis in many cases
- When available, World Health Organization (WHO) standards, or standards that can be linked to the WHO standard, should be used to calibrate funtional and antigenic assays
- Effect of age and sex should always be taken into consideration when interpreting the results of antigenic and functional assays
- Before concluding that a patient has an inherited thrombophilia, diagnostic assays for function or antigen should be repeated after excluding acquired aetiologies of the defect

### Further reading
- Cumming AM, Shiach CR. The investigation and management of inherited thrombophilia. *Clin Lab Haem* 1999;21:77-92
- Monagle P, Michelson AD, Bovill E, Andrew M. Antithrombotic therapy in children. *Chest* 2001;119:S344-70
- Streif W, Mitchell LG, Andrew M. Antithrombotic therapy in children. *Curr Opin Pediatr* 1999;11:56-64
- Haemostasis and Thrombosis Task Force, British Committee for Standards in Haematology. Guideline: investigation and management of heritable thrombophilia. *Br J Haematol* 2001;114:512-28

# 16   Anticoagulation in hospitals and general practice

Andrew D Blann, David A Fitzmaurice, Gregory Y H Lip

Service requirements for warfarin management include phlebotomy or finger pricking, accurate measurement of the international normalised ratio (INR) by a coagulometer (with associated standards and quality control), interpretation of the result, and advice on the warfarin dose. Clinical management of the complications of treatment (predominantly overdose) are also required. Furthermore, almost any drug can interact with oral anticoagulants, and many (such as steroids and antibiotics) often increase the anticoagulant effect.

When introducing a new drug, if the duration of treatment is short (such as an antibiotic for less than five days), then adjustment of dose is often not essential. If, however, the treatment is to last more than five days, then the INR should be checked after starting treatment with the new drug and the warfarin dose adjusted on the basis of the results.

1 mg (BROWN)

3 mg (BLUE)

5 mg (PINK)

Warfarin tablets used routinely in the United Kingdom

## Starting treatment in hospital inpatients

Once the indications for anticoagulation have been confirmed (for example, for suspected deep vein thrombosis do venography or D-dimer measurement), the initial dose of oral anticoagulant depends on a patient's coagulation status, age, clinical situation, and degree of heart failure (if present). In older patients, those with impaired liver function, and those with congestive heart failure oral anticoagulation should be started cautiously and the resulting INR checked often (every three to five days). The dose of warfarin needed to maintain an INR at 2.0-3.0, for example, falls with age and is greater in patients of Indo-Asian or African origin than in Europeans. Where possible, take routine blood samples for prothrombin time and activated partial thromboplastin time (APTT), platelet count, and liver function tests before starting treatment. Oral anticoagulation with warfarin should be started on day one, preferably in conjunction with heparin because the initial period of treatment with warfarin may be associated with a procoagulant state caused by a rapid reduction in protein C concentration (itself a vitamin K dependent protein). Heparin should not be stopped until the INR has been in the therapeutic range for two consecutive days. Patients at a high risk of thrombosis and those with a large atrial thrombus may need longer treatment with heparin.

Similarly, a specific anticoagulant treatment chart that contains the treatment protocol, the results of coagulation tests (INR and APTT ratios), and the prescribed doses based on the results should be the basis of treatment and is a useful way of assessing and monitoring patients' anticoagulation in the follow up period. Daily INR measurement for at least four days is recommended in patients needing rapid anticoagulation (for example, in those with high risk of thrombosis). Adjustment of the oral anticoagulant loading dose may be necessary if baseline coagulation results are abnormal. Some patients may be particularly sensitive to warfarin, such as older people and those with liver disease, congestive cardiac failure, or who are recieving drug treatment (such as antibiotics) likely to increase the effects of oral anticoagulants.

Once the therapeutic INR range is achieved it should be monitored weekly until control is stable. The British Society for Haematology's guidelines suggest that thereafter blood testing can be extended to fortnightly checks, then checks every four

---

**Drug interactions with warfarin***

*Enhanced anticoagulant effect*—Alcohol, allopurinol, anabolic steroids, analgesics (for example, paracetamol), antiarrhythmics (for example, amiodarone), antidepressants (for example, selective serotonin reuptake inhibitors), antidiabetics, antimalarials, antiplatelets, anxiolytics, disulfiram, influenza vaccine, leukotriene antagonists, levothyroxine, lipid regulating agents, testosterone, uricosurics

*Reduced anticoagulant effect*—Oral contraceptives, raloxifene, retinoids, rowachol, vitamin K (possibly present in enteral feeds)

*Variable effect*—Antibiotics (but, generally, more likely to enhance), colestyramine, antiepileptics, antifungals, barbiturates, cytotoxics (for example, effect enhanced by ifosfamide but often reduced by azathioprine), hormone antagonists, ulcer healing drugs

*This list is not exhaustive or definitive but provides perspective: the effect of each particular agent should be observed on each particular patient. Considerable variation exists in different drugs within a single class (for example, antibiotics). Refer to the *BNF* for guidance

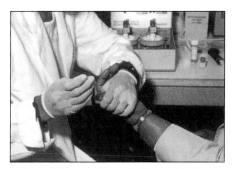

Anticoagulation monitoring by fingerprick. Note coagulometer in the background

weeks, eight weeks, and 12 weeks (maximum). By this time, the checks are most likely to be in the setting of an experienced hospital outpatient clinic.

At the time of discharge from hospital, follow up arrangements for each patient should include sufficient tablets to allow adequate cover until the general practitioner can provide a prescription (two to three weeks' worth) and an appointment for further INR measurements, generally in an outpatient clinic. This period should not exceed seven days and should be detailed in the patient case notes and the yellow Department of Health anticoagulant booklets. Information in the yellow booklet should indicate the target INR range for each patient and other pertinent information, such as the presence of diabetes and indication for anticoagulation.

## Starting treatment in outpatients

Without the benefit of the management procedures described above, starting anticoagulant treatment in outpatients can be difficult, especially if patients are referred without their notes or adequate information (such as other drugs prescribed or reason for anticoagulation). Nevertheless, local conditions and guidelines will generally recommend a starting dose, and patients will need to be recalled weekly for INR management until they are deemed to be stable. In many cases the introduction of computer assisted dosing (an algorithm software) is of immense benefit.

## Complications and reversal of oral anticoagulation

Bleeding complications while patients are receiving oral anticoagulants increase substantially when INR levels exceed 5.0, and therapeutic decisions depend on the presence of minor or major bleeding. However, in those cases with evidence of severe bleeding or haemodynamic compromise, hospitalisation, intensive monitoring, and resuscitation with intravenous fluids may be needed. Sometimes the bleeding point can be treated (for example, endoscopic treatment of bleeding peptic ulcer). Fresh frozen plasma is recommended when quick reversal of over-anticoagulation is needed. If plasma is unavailable then vitamin K, given by slow intravenous injection at doses of 0.5-1.0 mg or orally at doses of 1-10 mg, may reduce the INR within six to eight hours without the risk of over-correction. However, the effects of vitamin K can last for a week and may delay the restarting of warfarin treatment, although retesting (thus restarting with warfarin) after 48-72 hours is common.

## Maintenance in hospital practice

The traditional model of care for patients taking oral anticoagulants requires them to attend a hospital outpatient clinic so that the INR can be estimated. Capillary or venous blood samples are used, with the result being available either immediately or at a later stage. However, the INR derived from capillary (finger prick) blood is likely to be different from that obtained from plasma from a peripheral blood sample, and this should be considered. If possible, it is preferable to use consistently either finger prick or venous blood. Rarely, phlebotomists will visit housebound patients and return a venous sample to the laboratory for INR management. Where INR results are available with the patient present, dosing recommendations are made and the patient is given a date for the next appointment. When there is a delay in the INR estimation, patients receive dosing and recall advice through the

**Requirement for daily dose of warfarin to maintain an INR between 2.0 and 3.0 and 3.0 and 4.5**

| Age (years) | No of patients | Daily dose of warfarin (mg)* |
|---|---|---|
| INR to be in range 2.0 to 3.0 | | |
| 40-49 | 36 | 7.3 (6.21 to 8.39) |
| 50-59 | 76 | 5.5 (5.0 to 6.0) |
| 60-69 | 209 | 4.3 (4.05 to 4.55) |
| 70-79 | 233 | 3.9 (3.68 to 4.12) |
| ≥80 | 107 | 3.3 (3.01 to 3.59) |
| INR to be in range 3.0 to 4.5 | | |
| 40-49 | 9 | 6.5 (5.23 to 7.77) |
| 50-59 | 20 | 6.0 (5.2 to 6.8) |
| 60-69 | 45 | 5.9 (5.13 to 6.67) |
| 70-79 | 24 | 4.8 (4.15 to 5.45) |
| ≥80 | 2 | 4.2 (2.65 to 5.75) |

*Data are presented as mean (95% CI)
Relationship between age and daily dose in INR range 2.0-3.0 is correlation coefficient r = − 0.45, P < 0.001, and for INR range 3.0-4.5 is correlation coefficient r = − 0.23, P = 0.022
Data from Blann AD, et al, *Br J Haematol* 1999;107:207-9

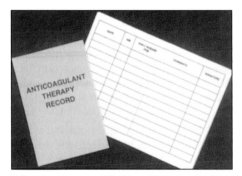

Yellow Department of Health anticoagulant booklet. Columns are provided for the date of each visit, INR result, recommended daily dose, and signature

**Treatment of excessive antithrombotic therapy effects**

| Class | Drug | Antidote |
|---|---|---|
| Oral anticoagulants | Warfarin | Oral or intravenous vitamin K; clotting factors or fresh frozen plasma, or both; recombinant factor VII |
| Intravenous or subdermal anticoagulants | Heparin | Protamine; clotting factors or fresh frozen plasma, or both |
| Thrombolytics | Streptokinase, tissue plasminogen activator (examples) | Transexamic acid |

post or by telephone. Although this service has been traditionally led by a physician (usually a consultant haematologist) or pathologist, more recently biomedical scientists, nurse specialists, and pharmacists have been taking responsibility for anticoagulant clinics. This model has been widely used in the United Kingdom but has come under more strain because of increasing numbers of patients referred for warfarin treatment, particularly for stroke prophylaxis in atrial fibrillation. However, in terms of INR control, adverse events, or patient satisfaction, long term oral anticoagulant care has traditionally required patients to attend a hospital anticoagulant clinic repeatedly because of the need for laboratory testing, specialist interpretation of the result, and adjustment of warfarin dose.

# Anticoagulation in general practice

Concerns over general practice involvement in anticoagulation monitoring have been expressed—namely, lack of resources (machines and reagents to generate the INR) and lack of expertise (experience and training), although these can be overcome. Despite various moves to decentralisation, no large scale development in a primary care setting has occurred. Understandably, general practitioners are anxious that decentralisation of anticoagulation care represents an additional, unwanted, and possibly dangerous burden. Local circumstances vary enormously so the process of decentralisation will need to be modified according to local needs and resources.

The establishment of a local development group consisting of general practitioners and hospital clinicians responsible for the anticoagulant clinic is one way of promoting decentralisation and identifying problem areas. There is increasing evidence that general practitioners or healthcare professionals such as biomedical scientists, pharmacists, and practice nurses, with or without computer assisted dosing, are able to achieve high standards of anticoagulation care with "near patient" testing. As the principle of near patient testing is well developed in glucose monitoring by or for diabetic patients, it seems logical that it can be transferred to oral anticoagulation, provided that adequate levels of accuracy and safety are achievable.

In one of the more widespread models general practitioners take a blood sample and dosing decisions are made by a hospital department, with patients receiving dosing information through the post or by telephone. This model retains the expertise and quality assurance of the laboratory process while decentralising at minimal cost to primary care. Patients can attend their (usually more convenient) general practitioner's surgery and a venous blood sample is sent to the central laboratory. INR is determined and information on dose and the next appointment is sent to the patient. There are no clinically significant changes in the INR when analysis is delayed for up to three days, and the quality control with near patient sampling is at least equal to that in a hospital based setting. This process requires access to phlebotomy in general practice, and the cost of testing and dosing remains in the central laboratory.

General practices with limited access to hospital clinics are more likely to undertake the second level of care and give dosing advice. General practitioners who do not have access to computer assisted dosing seem to have similar success to hospital clinics in achieving optimum INR control.

The third level of care uses near patient testing for INR estimation and computer assisted dosing for recommendation of dose and recall. Anticoagulant clinics are managed by practice nurses with support from the general practitioner and hospital laboratory. Liaison with the hospital laboratory is

---

**Factors affecting delivery of anticoagulation therapy**

**Hospital anticoagulation clinics**
- Usually busy and congested
- Congestion is an increasing problem caused by the ageing population with more indications for warfarin (especially atrial fibrillation)
- Inconvenient

**Domiciliary anticoagulation service**
- Depends on resources
- Limited availability
- Useful for those who are immobile or housebound

**"Near patient" testing**
- Requires considerable resources
- Dependent on primary care, facilities, and training

---

**Potential levels of involvement in general practice for managing anticoagulation treatment**

- Phlebotomy in the practice (by practice or hospital staff), blood sent (post or van) to the hospital laboratory with the result returned to the practice (telephone, fax, post, or email), dosing decisions being made in the practice, then communicated to the patient
- Phlebotomy in the practice, blood sent (post or van) to the hospital laboratory, dosing with INR estimation performed in the hospital and patient managed directly (telephone or post)
- Phlebotomy, INR estimation (plus dosing) and management all performed in the practice with hospital equipment and by hospital staff
- Phlebotomy, INR estimation plus dosing and management made by the practice (that is, full near patient testing); minimal input from the hospital

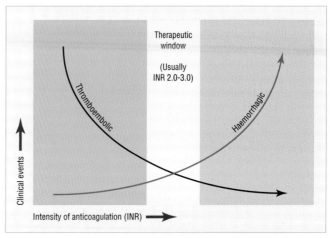

The therapeutic "window" is a balance between the best reduction in thromboembolic events and increased risk of bleeding with higher intensities of anticoagulation. Adapted from Hylek EM, et al. *New Engl J Med* 1993;120:897-902

paramount to the success of such a clinic as it needs to provide training and guidance on near patient testing technique, quality assurance, and health and safety issues. In a study by Fitzmaurice, et al (2000), INR therapeutic range analyses as point prevalence, proportion of tests in range, number of serious adverse events, and proportion of time in range all compared well with the hospital control patients. However, the proportion of time spent in the INR range showed substantial improvement for patients in the intervention group.

Computer assisted dosing aids interpretation of results, although it can be over-ridden if the suggestion made is not clinically indicated. For an effective and reliable service it is essential to ensure formal training and quality assurance procedures for near patient testing at the initial stages of the clinic development. This model of care gives an immediately available result, and, with close liaison with a hospital laboratory, it offers patients a complete model of care that would be a useful alternative to traditional care.

Another primary care model that has had limited evaluation is that of anticoagulant clinics that are managed entirely by scientists and pharmacists. These specialist healthcare professionals make use of their expertise in coagulation and pharmacology respectively. Secondary care anticoagulant clinics run by scientists and pharmacists have existed in the United Kingdom since 1979, and in terms of INR control they perform as well as clinics run by pathologists. Patients also prefer general practice management and welcome reduced waiting times and travelling costs. Improved patient understanding may also occur, which can help compliance. Further clinics managed by scientists or pharmacists, or both, are currently being evaluated.

## Patient self monitoring and dosing

Diabetic patients have long been able to use portable monitoring machines to check their own blood glucose concentrations and administer insulin accordingly. As equivalent machines for checking INR are now available, increased patient demand is likely to rise. The machine will appeal especially to those receiving long term anticoagulation whose lifestyle is not suited to the inconvenience of attending outpatient clinics. As with diabetic patients, well trained and motivated patients can probably attain a level of control of their own warfarin dose similar to that of the hospital. As yet, there are no comparison data on the safety and reliability of such an approach, so great caution is needed in offering (or even recommending) this option, which will be applicable to a well defined subset of patients. However, most pilot data suggest that patient self management is as safe as primary care management for a selected population, and further study is needed to show if this model of care is suitable for a larger population.

## Conclusion

The quality of anticoagulant care has improved in recent years with the development of clinical guidelines (for example, by the haemostasis and thrombosis task force of the British Society for Haematology), adoption of the INR system, quality control assurance, computerised decision support systems, and clinical audit. This allows a gradual movement of dosing from hospital to general practice. New models of delivering care (such as near patient testing) are now being developed to meet the increasing demand from an ageing population, such as from the growing number of patients with atrial fibrillation, whose risk of stroke is markedly reduced by anticoagulant therapy.

## Contraindications to warfarin use and management

**The patient**
- Comorbidity—including comorbid medical conditions, falls, frailty, exposure to trauma
- Impaired cognitive function
- Possibly housebound
- Poor compliance

**The doctor**
- Poor appreciation of drug interactions
- Inefficient organisation of INR monitoring

**The system**
- General practice v hospital facilities—for example remote location and poor communication and support
- Inadequate resources and facilities available

### Further reading

- Baglin T, Luddington R. Reliability of delayed INR determination: implications for decentralised anticoagulant care with off-site blood sampling. *Br J Haematol* 1997;96:431-4
- Blann AD, Hewitt J, Siddique F, Bareford D. Racial background is a determinant of average warfarin dose required to maintain the INR between 2.0 and 3.0. *Br J Haematol* 1999;107:207-9
- Fitzmaurice DA, Hobbs FDR, Delaney BC, Wilson S, McManus R. Review of computerized decision support systems for oral anticoagulation management. *Br J Haematol* 1998;102:907-9
- Fitzmaurice DA, Murray ET, Gee KM, Allan TF, Hobbs FD. A randomised controlled trial of patient self management of oral anticoagulation treatment compared with primary care management. *J Clin Pathol* 2002;55:845-9
- Fitzmaurice DA, Hobbs FD, Murray ET, Holder RL, Allan TF, Rose PE. Oral anticoagulation management in primary care with the use of computerized decision support and near-patient testing: a randomized, controlled trial. *Arch Intern Med* 2000;160:2343-8
- Haemostasis and Thrombosis Task Force of the British Society for Haematology. Guidelines on anticoagulation: third edition. *Br J Haematol* 1998;101:374-87
- MacGregor SH, Hamley JG, Dunbar JA, Dodd TRP, Cromarty JA. Evaluation of a primary care anticoagulation clinic managed by a pharmacist. *BMJ* 1996;312:560
- Pell JP, McIver B, Stuart P, Malone DNS, Alcock J. Comparison of anticoagulant control among patients attending general practice and a hospital anticoagulant clinic. *Br J Gen Pract* 1993;43:152-4
- Radley AS, Hall J, Farrow M, Carey PJ, Evaluation of anticoagulant control in a pharmacist operated anticoagulant clinic. *J Clin Pathol* 1995;48:545-7

# Index

Page numbers in **bold** type refer to figures; those in *italic* refer to tables or boxed material.

# Index

# Index